**HEALTH CARE ISSUES, COSTS AND ACCESS**

# U.S. MENTAL HEALTH WORKFORCE AND THE STATE OF THE MENTAL HEALTH SYSTEM

## A PRIMER AND PERSPECTIVES

# HEALTH CARE ISSUES, COSTS AND ACCESS

Additional books in this series can be found on Nova's website under the Series tab.

Additional e-books in this series can be found on Nova's website under the e-book tab.

HEALTH CARE ISSUES, COSTS AND ACCESS

# U.S. MENTAL HEALTH WORKFORCE AND THE STATE OF THE MENTAL HEALTH SYSTEM

# A PRIMER AND PERSPECTIVES

MAURICE GORDON
EDITOR

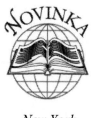

New York

Copyright © 2014 by Nova Science Publishers, Inc.

**All rights reserved.** No part of this book may be reproduced, stored in a retrieval system or transmitted in any form or by any means: electronic, electrostatic, magnetic, tape, mechanical photocopying, recording or otherwise without the written permission of the Publisher.

For permission to use material from this book please contact us:
Telephone 631-231-7269; Fax 631-231-8175
Web Site: http://www.novapublishers.com

## NOTICE TO THE READER

The Publisher has taken reasonable care in the preparation of this book, but makes no expressed or implied warranty of any kind and assumes no responsibility for any errors or omissions. No liability is assumed for incidental or consequential damages in connection with or arising out of information contained in this book. The Publisher shall not be liable for any special, consequential, or exemplary damages resulting, in whole or in part, from the readers' use of, or reliance upon, this material. Any parts of this book based on government reports are so indicated and copyright is claimed for those parts to the extent applicable to compilations of such works.

Independent verification should be sought for any data, advice or recommendations contained in this book. In addition, no responsibility is assumed by the publisher for any injury and/or damage to persons or property arising from any methods, products, instructions, ideas or otherwise contained in this publication.

This publication is designed to provide accurate and authoritative information with regard to the subject matter covered herein. It is sold with the clear understanding that the Publisher is not engaged in rendering legal or any other professional services. If legal or any other expert assistance is required, the services of a competent person should be sought. FROM A DECLARATION OF PARTICIPANTS JOINTLY ADOPTED BY A COMMITTEE OF THE AMERICAN BAR ASSOCIATION AND A COMMITTEE OF PUBLISHERS.

Additional color graphics may be available in the e-book version of this book.

**LIBRARY OF CONGRESS CATALOGING-IN-PUBLICATION DATA**

ISBN: 978-1-62948-865-3

*Published by Nova Science Publishers, Inc. † New York*

# CONTENTS

| | | |
|---|---|---|
| **Preface** | | vii |
| **Chapter 1** | The Mental Health Workforce: A Primer<br>*Elayne J. Heisler and Erin Bagalman* | 1 |
| **Chapter 2** | Statement of Pamela S. Hyde, Administrator, Substance Abuse and Mental Health Services Administration. Hearing on "Assessing the State of America's Mental Health System" | 27 |
| **Chapter 3** | Testimony of Thomas Insel, Director, National Institute of Mental Health. Hearing on "Assessing the State of America's Mental Health System" | 39 |
| **Chapter 4** | Testimony of Michael F. Hogan, Former Commissioner, New York State Office of Mental Health. Hearing on "Assessing the State of America's Mental Health System" | 45 |
| **Chapter 5** | Testimony of Dr. Bob Vero, CEO, Centerstone of Tennessee. Hearing on "Assessing the State of America's Mental Health System" | 55 |
| **Chapter 6** | Testimony of Larry Fricks, Senior Consultant, National Council for Community Behavioral Healthcare. Hearing on "Assessing the State of America's Mental Health System" | 67 |

| | | |
|---|---|---|
| **Chapter 7** | Testimony of George DelGrosso, Executive Director, Colorado Behavioral Health Council. Hearing on "Assessing the State of America's Mental Health System" | 73 |
| **Chapter 8** | Testimony of Robert Petzel, Under Secretary for Health, Veterans Health Administration, Department of Veterans Affairs. Hearing on ''VA Mental Health Care: Ensuring Timely Access to High-Quality Care" | 77 |
| **Chapter 9** | Statement of Pamela S. Hyde, Administrator, Substance Abuse and Mental Health Services Administration. Hearing on "Examining SAMHSA's Role in Delivering Services to the Severely Mentally Ill" | 97 |
| **Index** | | 113 |

# PREFACE

The federal government is involved in mental health care in various ways, including direct provision of services, payment for services, and indirect support for services. Policy makers have demonstrated interest in the federal government's broad role in mental health care. They have done so primarily by holding hearings and introducing legislation addressing the interrelated topics of quality of mental health care, access to mental health care, and the cost of mental health care. This book begins with a working definition of the mental health workforce and a brief discussion of alternative definitions. It then describes three dimensions of the mental health workforce that may influence quality of care, access to care, and costs of care. The book then briefly discusses how these dimensions of the mental health workforce might inform certain policy discussions, and provides statements and testimonies from various individuals on mental health care.

Chapter 1 - Congress has held hearings and introduced legislation addressing the interrelated topics of the quality of mental health care, access to mental health care, and the cost of mental health care. The mental health workforce is a key component of each of these topics. The quality of mental health care depends partially on the skills of the people providing the care. Access to mental health care relies on, among other things, the number of appropriately skilled providers available to provide care. The cost of mental health care depends in part on the wages of the people providing care. Thus an understanding of the mental health workforce may be helpful in crafting policy and conducting oversight. This report aims to provide such an understanding as a foundation for further discussion of mental health policy.

No consensus exists on which provider types make up the mental health workforce. This report focuses on the five provider types identified by the

Health Resources and Services Administration (HRSA) within the Department of Health and Human Services (HHS) as "core mental health professionals": psychiatrists, clinical psychologists, clinical social workers, advanced practice psychiatric nurses, and marriage and family therapists. The HRSA definition of the mental health workforce is limited to highly trained (e.g., graduate degree) professionals; however, this workforce may be defined more broadly elsewhere.

An understanding of typical licensure requirements and scopes of practice may help policy makers determine how to focus policy initiatives aimed at increasing the quality of the mental health workforce. Although state licensure requirements vary widely across provider types, the scopes of practice converge into provider types that generally can prescribe medication (psychiatrists and advanced practice psychiatric nurses) and provider types that generally cannot prescribe medication (clinical psychologists, clinical social workers, and marriage and family therapists). The core mental health provider types can all provide psychosocial interventions (e.g., talk therapy). Administration and interpretation of psychological tests is generally the province of clinical psychologists.

Access to mental health care depends in part on the number of mental health providers overall and the number of specific types of providers. Clinical social workers are generally the most plentiful core mental health provider type, followed by clinical psychologists, who substantially outnumber marriage and family therapists. While less abundant than the three aforementioned provider types, psychiatrists outnumber advanced practice psychiatric nurses. Policy makers may influence the size of the mental health workforce through a number of health workforce training programs.

Policy makers may assess the relative wages of different provider types, particularly when addressing policy areas where the federal government employs mental health providers. Psychiatrists are the highest earners, followed by advanced practice psychiatric nurses and clinical psychologists. Marriage and family therapists earn more than clinical social workers. The relative costs of employing different provider types may be a consideration for federal agencies that employ mental health providers.

Chapter 2 - Statement of Pamela S. Hyde, Administrator, Substance Abuse and Mental Health Services Administration.

Chapter 3 - Testimony of Thomas Insel, Director, National Institute of Mental Health.

Chapter 4 - Testimony of Michael F. Hogan, Former Commissioner, New York State Office of Mental Health.

Chapter 5 - Testimony of Dr. Bob Vero, CEO, Centerstone of Tennessee.

Chapter 6 - Testimony of Larry Fricks, Senior Consultant, National Council for Community Behavioral Healthcare.

Chapter 7 - Testimony of George DelGrosso, Executive Director, Colorado Behavioral Health Council.

Chapter 8 - Testimony of Robert Petzel, Under Secretary for Health, Veterans Health Administration, Department of Veterans Affairs.

Chapter 9 - Statement of Pamela S. Hyde, Administrator, Substance Abuse and Mental Health Services Administration.

In: U.S. Mental Health Workforce ...
Editor: Maurice Gordon

ISBN: 978-1-62948-865-3
© 2014 Nova Science Publishers, Inc.

*Chapter 1*

# THE MENTAL HEALTH WORKFORCE: A PRIMER[*]

## *Elayne J. Heisler and Erin Bagalman*

### SUMMARY

Congress has held hearings and introduced legislation addressing the interrelated topics of the quality of mental health care, access to mental health care, and the cost of mental health care. The mental health workforce is a key component of each of these topics. The quality of mental health care depends partially on the skills of the people providing the care. Access to mental health care relies on, among other things, the number of appropriately skilled providers available to provide care. The cost of mental health care depends in part on the wages of the people providing care. Thus an understanding of the mental health workforce may be helpful in crafting policy and conducting oversight. This report aims to provide such an understanding as a foundation for further discussion of mental health policy.

No consensus exists on which provider types make up the mental health workforce. This report focuses on the five provider types identified by the Health Resources and Services Administration (HRSA) within the Department of Health and Human Services (HHS) as "core mental health professionals": psychiatrists, clinical psychologists, clinical social

---

[*] This is an edited, reformatted and augmented version of a Congressional Research Service publication, CRS Report for Congress R43255, prepared for Members and Committees of Congress, from www.crs.gov, dated October 18, 2013.

workers, advanced practice psychiatric nurses, and marriage and family therapists. The HRSA definition of the mental health workforce is limited to highly trained (e.g., graduate degree) professionals; however, this workforce may be defined more broadly elsewhere.

An understanding of typical licensure requirements and scopes of practice may help policy makers determine how to focus policy initiatives aimed at increasing the quality of the mental health workforce. Although state licensure requirements vary widely across provider types, the scopes of practice converge into provider types that generally can prescribe medication (psychiatrists and advanced practice psychiatric nurses) and provider types that generally cannot prescribe medication (clinical psychologists, clinical social workers, and marriage and family therapists). The core mental health provider types can all provide psychosocial interventions (e.g., talk therapy). Administration and interpretation of psychological tests is generally the province of clinical psychologists.

Access to mental health care depends in part on the number of mental health providers overall and the number of specific types of providers. Clinical social workers are generally the most plentiful core mental health provider type, followed by clinical psychologists, who substantially outnumber marriage and family therapists. While less abundant than the three aforementioned provider types, psychiatrists outnumber advanced practice psychiatric nurses. Policy makers may influence the size of the mental health workforce through a number of health workforce training programs.

Policy makers may assess the relative wages of different provider types, particularly when addressing policy areas where the federal government employs mental health providers. Psychiatrists are the highest earners, followed by advanced practice psychiatric nurses and clinical psychologists. Marriage and family therapists earn more than clinical social workers. The relative costs of employing different provider types may be a consideration for federal agencies that employ mental health providers.

# INTRODUCTION

The federal government is involved in mental health care in various ways, including direct provision of services, payment for services, and indirect support for services (e.g., grant funding, dissemination of best practices, and technical assistance).[1] Policy makers have demonstrated interest in the federal government's broad role in mental health care. They have done so primarily by holding hearings[2] and introducing legislation[3] addressing the interrelated topics of quality of mental health care, access to mental health care, and the cost of mental health care.

The mental health workforce is a key component of mental health care quality, access, and cost. The quality of mental health care, for example, is influenced by the skills of the people providing the care. Access to mental health care depends on the number of appropriately skilled providers available to provide care, among other things. The cost of mental health care is affected in part by the wages of the people providing care. Thus an understanding of the mental health workforce may be helpful in crafting legislation and conducting oversight for overall mental health care policy.

It is important to note that, while the federal government has an interest in the mental health workforce, and federal initiatives may affect the training of mental health care providers, for instance, most of the regulation of the mental health workforce occurs at the state level. State boards determine licensing requirements for mental health professionals, and state laws establish their scopes of practice.

This report begins with a working definition of the mental health workforce and a brief discussion of alternative definitions. It then describes three dimensions of the mental health workforce that may influence quality of care, access to care, and costs of care: (1) licensure requirements and scope of practice for each provider type in the mental health workforce, (2) estimated numbers of each provider type in the mental health workforce, and (3) average annual wages for each provider type in the mental health workforce. The report then briefly discusses how these dimensions of the mental health workforce might inform certain policy discussions.

## **MENTAL HEALTH WORKFORCE DEFINITION: NO CONSENSUS**

No consensus exists on which provider types make up the mental health workforce. While some define the workforce as a broad range of provider types, others take a more narrow approach. For example, the Institute of Medicine (IOM)—a private, nonprofit organization that aims to provide evidence-based health policy advice to decision makers, often through congressionally mandated studies—has conceptualized the mental health workforce broadly, including primary care physicians, nurses, physician assistants, peer support specialists, and family caregivers, among others.[4] The

Substance Abuse and Mental Health Services Administration (SAMHSA)—the public health agency within the Department of Health and Human Services (HHS) that leads efforts to improve the nation's mental health—has in recent years defined the mental health workforce to include psychiatry, clinical psychology, clinical social work, advanced practice psychiatric nursing, marriage and family therapy, and counseling.[5] In the past, SAMSHA's mental health workforce definition has also included psychosocial rehabilitation, school psychology, and pastoral counseling.[6]

The Health Resources and Services Administration (HRSA)—the public health agency within HHS with primary responsibility for increasing access to health care (including mental health care) for vulnerable populations[7]—provides a more narrow definition of the mental health workforce that is tied to existing federal programs aimed at alleviating provider shortages (e.g., Medicare bonus payments and health workforce recruitment programs). Eligibility for such programs is determined in part by the designation of a Mental Health Professional Shortage Area (MHPSA).[8] The MHPSA designation is based on a limited number of core provider types because it is intended to identify the most extreme workforce shortages in order to target federal investments. For purposes of designating MHPSAs, HRSA identifies "[c]ore mental health professionals [as] psychiatrists, clinical psychologists, clinical social workers, [advanced practice psychiatric nurses],[9] and marriage and family therapists" who meet specified training and licensing criteria (as detailed in *Appendix A*). Notably, this definition is limited to highly trained mental health professionals.

## MENTAL HEALTH WORKFORCE OVERVIEW

In conceptualizing and outlining the mental health workforce, this report relies on the HRSA definition of "core mental health professionals," including psychiatrists, clinical psychologists, clinical social workers, advanced practice psychiatric nurses, and marriage and family therapists.[10] For each of the five core mental health professions, *Table 1* summarizes licensure requirements (including degree, supervised practice, and exam) and scope of practice; each of these terms is explained briefly below. Although the licensure requirements vary widely across provider types, the scopes of practice converge into provider types that generally can prescribe medication (psychiatrists and advanced practice psychiatric nurses) and provider types that generally cannot prescribe medication (clinical psychologists, clinical social workers, and marriage and family therapists). All provider types in this report can provide psychosocial interventions (e.g., talk therapy). Administration and interpretation of psychological tests is generally the province of clinical psychologists.

## Licensure Requirements

Licensure requirements are the minimum qualifications needed to obtain and maintain a license in a specific health profession. These requirements are generally defined by state licensing boards— independent entities to which state governments have delegated the authority to set licensure requirements for specified professions. State licensing boards generally have responsibility for verifying that requirements to obtain (and maintain) a license have been met, issuing initial and renewed licenses, and tracking licensure violations, among other activities.[11]

*Table 1* focuses on licensure requirements that are common across many states; it generally does not address state variation. Across all provider types, the table addresses licensure for independent clinical practice,[12] although some disciplines offer licensing at lower practice levels or provisional licensing. The table describes requirements to *obtain* a license and does not include requirements to *maintain* a license (e.g., continuing education).[13]

### *Degree*

The degree noted in *Table 1* indicates the minimum level of education generally required to be licensed for independent practice.[14] For the core mental health professionals outlined in this report, licensure for independent practice requires the completion of graduate education.[15] *Table 1* generally does not include degrees that are prerequisites for graduate education (e.g., a bachelor's degree) or degrees beyond those required for licensure (e.g., a doctoral degree available in a discipline where a master's degree is qualifying for licensure for independent practice). Notably, in order to enroll in a graduate program to become an advanced practice psychiatric nurse, an individual must first be a *registered nurse* with a bachelor's degree in nursing. The other provider types in this report do not have equivalent requirements for specific undergraduate degrees or for prior licensing.

*Table 1* provides a brief description of each graduate degree, including requirements such as a field experience or a dissertation. The table also indicates the amount of time typically required to complete the degree. In some cases, individuals may complete the degree in less time (e.g., by participating in an accelerated program) or more time (e.g., by attending school part-time or taking longer to complete a dissertation).

### *Supervised Practice*

For most provider types discussed in this report, licensure for independent practice requires a period of post-graduate supervised practice. This period of supervised practice is distinct from the practicum or internship experiences required to obtain a degree.

An example of such supervised practice is the residency required for physicians to become psychiatrists.

### *Exam*

State licensing boards generally require a passing score on an exam offered by a national body (e.g., the American Board of Psychiatry and Neurology), although some state licensing boards may offer their own exams in addition to or in lieu of the national exam. In some cases, individuals applying for licensure may have a choice of exams that meet the licensure requirement. The timing of the exam may vary by state; that is, some states may allow individuals to take the exam immediately upon completing the degree requirements, while other states may require individuals to have completed a portion (or all) of the supervised practice requirement prior to taking the exam.

## Scope of Practice

The scope of practice for each provider type is established at the state level by state statute, regulation, or guidance. *Table 1* highlights elements within scope of practice that involve *diagnosing* and *treating* mental illness. The scope of practice for most provider types includes other activities, such as preventive care, case management, and consultation with other providers. The scope of practice described in the table reflects what is generally true in most states.

For example, prescribing medication is included in the scope of practice for advanced practice psychiatric nurses, a provider type that comprises both nurse practitioners (allowed to prescribe medication in all states) and clinical nurse specialists (allowed to prescribe medication in only some states).

**Table 1. Licensure Requirements and Scope of Practice, by Mental Health Provider Type**

| Provider Type[a] | Licensure Requirements | | | Scope of Practice[b] |
|---|---|---|---|---|
| | Degree[c] | Supervised Practice | Exam | |
| Psychiatrist | Medical Doctorate (MD) or Doctorate of Osteopathic Medicine (DO), both of which typically require 4 years to complete (including 2 years of clinical rotations). Coursework emphasizes physical medicine. | Generally requires 3 or 4 years of post-degree supervised clinical training (residency) in the specialty of psychiatry. | Generally requires a passing score on the United States Medical Licensing Examination (USMLE) for MDs or DOs.[d] DOs can also elect to take the Comprehensive Osteopathic Medical Licensing Examination (COMLEX). To become board certified, an exam administered by the American Board of Psychiatry and Neurology.[e] | • Diagnose mental disorders.<br>• Provide psychosocial treatment for individuals, families, and groups.<br>• Can prescribe medication.<br>• Can diagnose and treat physical conditions as well. |
| Clinical Psychologist | Doctoral degree in psychology or a related field, which generally takes between 5 and 7 years to complete and requires academic coursework, clinical training, a dissertation, and an exam. | Generally requires 3,000 hours of supervised clinical training, which take approximately 2 years.[f] | Generally requires a passing score on the Examination for Professional Practice in Psychology (EPPP).[g] | • Diagnose mental disorders.<br>• Provide psychosocial treatment for individuals, families, and groups.<br>• Administer and interpret psychological tests.<br>• Generally cannot prescribe medication.[h] |

## Table 1. (Continued)

| Provider Type[a] | Licensure Requirements | | | Scope of Practice[b] |
|---|---|---|---|---|
| | Degree[c] | Supervised Practice | Exam | |
| Clinical Social Worker | Master of Social Work (MSW), which typically requires 2 years. Coursework emphasizes human and community well-being. Requires a supervised field practicum (internship). | Generally requires 3,200–3,400 post-degree supervised clinical hours, which take approximately 2 years. | Generally requires a passing score on the Clinical Exam of the Association of Social Work Boards. | • Diagnose mental disorders.<br>• Provide psychosocial treatment for individuals, families, and groups.<br>• Cannot prescribe medication. |
| Advanced Practice Psychiatric Nurse (APPN)[i] | Master of Science (MS) in nursing, which generally requires 2 years of coursework and clinical hours (generally 500 or more).[j] Coursework and clinical experience focus on psychiatric mental health nursing. | No separate post-graduate clinical training is required. | As of January 1, 2014, will require a passing score on an exam offered by the American Nurses Credentialing Center.[k] | • Diagnose mental disorders.<br>• Provide psychosocial treatment for individuals, families, and groups.<br>• Generally can prescribe medication.<br>• Can diagnose and treat physical conditions as well.[l] |
| Marriage and Family Therapist (MFT) | Master's degree (2-3 years), doctoral degree (3-5 years), or postgraduate clinical training (3-4 years) in marriage and family therapy or a related field.[m] Coursework emphasizes the | Generally requires 2 years of post-degree supervised clinical training. | Generally requires a passing score on the Association of Marital and Family Therapy Regulatory Board's Examination in Marriage and Family or the equivalent California | • Diagnose mental disorders.<br>• Provide psychosocial treatment for individuals, families, and groups.<br>• Cannot prescribe medication. |

| Provider Type[a] | Licensure Requirements | | | Scope of Practice[b] |
|---|---|---|---|---|
| | Degree[c] | Supervised Practice | Exam | |
| | individual's mental health in the context of interpersonal relationships (e.g., family and peers). Generally requires a field practicum or internship. | | Exam.[n] | |

Source: U.S. Department of Labor, Bureau of Labor Statistics; U.S. Department of Health and Human Services, Health Resources and Services Administration (HRSA); and various professional associations. For more information on the professional organizations for each of five health professions, see Appendix B.

Notes: The degree, supervised practice, and exam indicated in the table are those generally required to obtain a license for independent practice. Licensure requirements (defined by state boards) and scope of practice (defined by state laws) vary by state.

Degree requirements may vary by program. In all cases, the information provided in the table reflects what is generally true in most states and programs. Elaborating the exceptions is beyond the scope of this report.

[a] The provider type may not correspond to the name of the license (which may vary by state for some provider types). The provider types correspond to HRSA's "core mental health professionals" (with the exception of advanced practice psychiatric nurses, which HRSA calls "psychiatric nurse specialists").

[b] The table focuses on the elements within scope of practice that involve diagnosing and treating mental illness. The scope of practice for most provider types includes other activities, such as preventive care, case management, and consultation with other providers.

[c] The table focuses on graduate degree requirements (i.e., post-baccalaureate training requirements).

[d] Graduates of certain foreign medical schools may also be eligible to take the USMLE.

[e] The term "board certified physician" means one who has completed the required training in a specific specialty and has passed an examination that assesses the basic knowledge and skills in a particular area (in this case psychiatry or neurology). Board certification is not required to practice as a psychiatrist but may be a condition of employment for some employers.

[f] Generally, states require that at least 1,500 hours (of the 3,000 hours required) be a post-doctoral experience. See Association of State and Provincial Psychology

Boards, "Entry Requirements for the Professional Practice of Psychology, 2008," http://www.asppb.net/files/public/09_Entry_Requirements.pdf.

[g] A board certified psychologist is one who has completed training in a specific specialty and has passed an examination that assesses the basic knowledge and skills in that particular area. As in psychiatry, board certification is not required, but some employers may require it. Board certification is conducted by the American Board of Professional Psychology, see http://www.abpp.org/.

[h] In New Mexico, Louisiana, Guam, the U.S. Department of Defense (DOD) system, the Indian Health Service, and the U.S. Public Health Service, licensed psychologists who obtain additional training can apply to have prescription writing privileges as part of their scope of practice. See Robert E. McGrath, "Prescriptive Authority for Psychologists," Annual Review of Clinical Psychology, vol. 6 (April 27, 2010), pp. 21-47.

[i] This includes mental health/psychiatric nurse practitioners and clinical nurse specialists. This report uses the term "advanced practice psychiatric nurse," which is more common than the term "psychiatric nurse specialists" used by HRSA. The American Psychiatric Nurses Association (APNA) aims to bring uniformity to the requirements for advanced practice psychiatric nurses by 2015, in accordance with the "Consensus Model for APRN Regulation:
Licensure, Accreditation, Certification & Education;" see American Psychiatric Nurses Association, APRN Consensus Model, http://www.apna.org/i4a/pages/index.cfm?pageID=4387.

[j] The nursing profession is moving towards requiring doctoral degrees in these fields, which requires an additional two years of training. See American Psychiatric Nurses Association, "What is an Advanced Practice Psychiatric Nurse?" http://www.apna.org/i4a/pages/index.cfm?pageID=3866.

[k] Until January 1, 2014, the American Nurses Credentialing Center offers four different exams: two for Nurse Practitioners (in Adult or Family Psychiatry) and two for Clinical Nurse Specialists (in Adult or Child/Adolescent Psychiatric Nursing). In order to become an advanced practice psychiatric nurse, an individual must first be a registered nurse, which generally requires a passing score on the National Council Licensure Examination-RN (NCLEX-RN). See National Council of State Boards of Nursing, NCLEX Examinations, https://www.ncsbn.org/nclex.htm.

[l] Some states may require that advanced practice psychiatric nurses be supervised by physicians.

[m] Related fields may include psychology, social work, nursing, education, or pastoral counseling. See American Association for Marriage and Family Therapy, About AAMFT, Qualifications and FAQs, http://www.aamft.org/imis15/content/about_aamft/Qualifications.aspx.

[n] Marriage and Family Therapists (MFTs) who practice in California (representing more n than half of all MFTs), must pass a separate California licensing exam.

## MENTAL HEALTH WORKFORCE SIZE

Access to mental health care depends in part on the overall number of practicing mental health providers and the number of specific types of providers.[16] As of June 2013, HRSA had designated 3,744 Mental Health Professional Shortage Areas (MHPSAs), including one or more in each state, the District of Columbia, and each of the territories.[17] Although HRSA designates MHPSAs, it does not collect data on the size of the mental health workforce nationally.[18] *Figure 1* and *Table 2* both present workforce size estimates for each core mental health provider type from

- The Mental Health and Substance Use Workforce for Older Adults: In Whose Hands? by the Institute of Medicine (IOM);[19]
- Mental Health, United States, 2010 by the Substance Abuse and Mental Health Services Administration (SAMHSA);[20] and
- other sources, including professional associations and licensing boards.

Although the number of mental health providers in each profession varies across the three sources, each source yields the same order of provider types from most plentiful to least plentiful, as illustrated in *Figure 1*. According to each data source, clinical social workers are estimated to be the most plentiful, followed by clinical psychologists, who substantially outnumber marriage and family therapists. While less abundant than the three aforementioned provider types, psychiatrists outnumber advanced practice psychiatric nurses.

Variation in the numbers from different sources reflects some of the difficulty in determining the size of the workforce—and therefore also in determining the adequacy of the workforce to provide access to mental health care. Along with workforce size estimates for each provider type, *Table 2* presents the *original* data sources (e.g., the IOM report relies primarily on data from the Bureau of Labor Statistics within the U.S. Department of Labor). Limitations of each original data source may lead to overstating or understating the number of providers (e.g., the Bureau of Labor Statistics data excludes self-employed workers). Major limitations are noted in *Table 2*.

Even looking at the numbers in relative terms, the limitations of the original sources complicate comparisons across professions. For example, the Bureau of Labor Statistics figures in the IOM report *include* school psychologists and *exclude* school social workers, limiting their comparability.

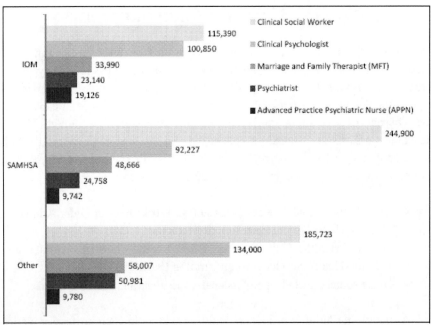

Source: CRS analysis of data from Institute of Medicine, The Mental Health and Substance use Workforce for Older Adults: In Whose Hands? (Washington, DC: National Academies Press, 2012); Substance Abuse and Mental Health Services Administration, Mental Health, United States, 2010, Rockville, MD, 2010; and other sources (i.e., professional associations and licensing boards).

Figure 1. Workforce Size Estimates, by Mental Health Provider Type.

**Table 2. Workforce Size Estimates, by Mental Health Provider Type**

| Provider Type | Institute of Medicine Report[a] | | Mental Health, United States, 2010[b] | | | Other Sources (Membership and Licensing) |
|---|---|---|---|---|---|---|
| Psychiatrist | 23,140 | BLS, May 2011, estimate of psychiatrists (SOC 29-1066). Excludes the self-employed. | 24,758 | American Psychiatric Association, 2006, membership. Excludes students, residents, fellows, international members, and inactive members. Not all psychiatrists are members. | 50,981 | American Medical Association, 2012, Board Certified Psychiatrists. Includes psychiatrists who are not practicing (e.g., researchers or retired). |
| Clinical Psychologist | 100,850 | BLS, May 2011, estimate of clinical, counseling, and | 92,227 | American Psychological Association, 2006, Member Directory. | 134,000 | American Psychological Association, 2013, members. Includes |

| Provider Type | Institute of Medicine Report[a] | | Mental Health, United States, 2010[b] | | | Other Sources (Membership and Licensing) |
|---|---|---|---|---|---|---|
| | | school psychologists (SOC 19-3031). Excludes the self-employed. | | Not all psychologists are members. | | members who are not mental health providers (e.g., experimental psychologists). Excludes non-members. |
| Clinical Social Worker | 115,390 | BLS, May 2011, estimate of mental health and substance abuse social workers (SOC 21-1023). Excludes the self-employed. | 244,900 | Calculated as 79% of the number of licensed social workers (per the Association of Social Work Boards), the estimated percent eligible to hold clinical licenses. | 185,723 | Association of Social Work Boards, Inc., 2011, sum of state-level numbers of MSWs with experience. May double-count those licensed in multiple states. Excludes those from states that did not report. |
| Advanced Practice Psychiatric Nurse (APPN) | 19,126 | National Sample Survey of Registered Nurses, 2008, estimates of psychiatric advanced practice registered nurses. | 9,742 | American Nurses Credentialing Center, 2006, Advanced Practice Psychiatric Nurses. | 9,780 | American Nurses Credentialing Center, 2008, sum of state-level numbers of APPNs.[c] May double-count those licensed in multiple states. |
| Marriage and Family Therapist (MFT) | 33,990 | BLS, May 2011, estimate of marriage and family therapists (SOC 21-1013). Excludes the self-employed. | 48,666 | American Association for Marriage and Family Therapy, 2006, Membership Database of clinical members. | 58,007 | American Association for Marriage and Family Therapy, 2013, sum of state-level numbers of fully licensed MFTs from state boards. May double-count those licensed in multiple states. Excludes those with provisional licenses. |

Notes: BLS = Bureau of Labor Statistics; SOC = Standard Occupational Classification (codes used by the Bureau of Labor Statistics).

[a] From Institute of Medicine. (2012). The Mental Health and Substance Use Workforce for Older Adults: In Whose Hands? Washington, DC: The National Academies Press. See Table 3-2 "Estimated Number of Mental Health/Substance Use (MH/SU) Specialists, 2011." For all provider types other than advanced practice psychiatric nurses, IOM used data from the Bureau of Labor Statistics (BLS), Occupational Employment Statistics, Occupational Employment and Wages, May 2011. BLS estimates are based on a survey that excludes self-employed workers.

[b] From Substance Abuse and Mental Health Services Administration. (2012). Mental Health, United States, 2010. HHS Publication No. (SMA) 12-4681. Rockville, MD: Substance Abuse and Mental Health Services Administration. See Table 45 "Number and percentage of clinically trained mental health personnel, by discipline and distribution, by sex, age, and Hispanic origin and race, United States, selected years."

[c] Cited in Hanrahan et al. (2010), "Health Care Reform and the Federal Transformation Initiatives: Capitalizing on the Potential of Advanced Practice Psychiatric Nurses," Policy, Politics, & Nursing Practice 11(3): 235-244.

## MENTAL HEALTH WORKFORCE ANNUAL WAGES

Just as access to mental health care providers depends partially on the size of the mental health workforce, the cost of mental health care depends partly on the wages paid to mental health providers. *Table 3* presents mean and median annual wages from the Bureau of Labor Statistics (BLS). These wage data are widely used because of their large sample size, broad geographic reach, and the comparable methodology used to collect data across occupations.[21] Information from BLS is likely to either over- or under-state wages for some mental health providers; the data are based on a survey that excludes self-employed workers (i.e., those in private practice), who may have different incomes. For example, for both clinical psychologists and clinical social workers, the categories used by the BLS include individuals who may earn substantially less than those who meet the HRSA definition of the provider type. The wage estimates for clinical psychologists are based on a category that includes school psychologists, who do not have to meet the same licensure requirements as HRSA-defined clinical psychologists and thus might receive lower wages. Similarly, the wage estimates for clinical social workers are based on a category that includes individuals who are not licensed for independent practice and who also might earn less.

Despite their limitations, the BLS data are able to illuminate the relative wages of each provider type as outlined in *Table 3*. Psychiatrists are the relative highest earners, followed by advanced practice psychiatric nurses and clinical psychologists. Marriage and family therapists generally earn more than clinical social workers.

### Table 3. Mean and Median Annual Wages, by Mental Health Provider Type

| Provider Type | Annual Wage | | BLS Category Used[a] |
|---|---|---|---|
| | Mean | Median | |
| Psychiatrist | $177,520 | $173,330 | Psychiatrists (SOC 29-1066). |
| Clinical Psychologist | $72,220 | $67,650 | Clinical, Counseling, and School Psychologists (SOC 19-3031). |
| Clinical Social Worker | $43,340 | $39,980 | Mental Health and Substance Abuse Social Workers (SOC 21-1023). No distinction is made between levels of education or licensure. |
| Advanced Practice Psychiatric Nurse (APPN) | $91,450 | $89,960 | Nurse Practitioners (SOC 29-1171). No estimate is provided for the psychiatric/mental health specialty. |
| Marriage and Family Therapist (MFT) | $49,270 | $46,670 | Marriage and Family Therapists (SOC 21-1013). |

Source: CRS summary of data from U.S. Department of Labor, Bureau of Labor Statistics, Occupational Employment Statistics, May 2012 Occupation Profiles, http://www.bls.gov/oes/current/oes_stru.htm.

[a] BLS wage estimates do not include self-employed workers. SOC = Standard Occupational Classification (codes used by the Bureau of Labor Statistics).

## CONCLUSION

Understanding the mental health workforce may help policy makers address a range of potential policy issues related to mental health care, including its quality, access, and cost.

An understanding of typical licensure requirements and scopes of practice may help policy makers determine how to direct federal policy initiatives focused on enhancing the quality of mental health care such as those related to training mental health providers. If, for example, training new providers quickly is a priority, initiatives may focus on training additional providers who can be licensed with a master's degree, rather than a doctoral degree. Initiatives may focus on training providers who can prescribe medication if the need is greater for medication than for psychosocial interventions. Going beyond the provider types discussed in this report, if a priority is to expand the breadth of the mental health workforce, policy makers might also consider federal training directed toward initiatives that focus on paraprofessionals who do not require extensive training or toward primary care professionals who do not specialize in mental health but may provide care for individuals with mental illness. Increasing the breadth of the mental health workforce may also increase its overall size.

Another way policy makers may influence the size of the mental health workforce (and thus access to mental health services) is through the provision or expansion of federal programs.[22] For example, the federal government may provide grants to establish or expand training programs for mental health providers. The federal government may also provide incentives such as loan repayment or loan forgiveness to encourage individuals to enter mental health occupations, which are projected to grow faster than the overall workforce.[23] Policy makers may consider strategies to direct people into these high growth fields as part of larger labor force policy considerations. Initiatives may be targeted to certain provider types or to certain locations (e.g., MHPSAs).

Policy makers may also wish to consider the relative wages of different provider types, particularly when addressing domains within which the federal government employs mental health providers. For instance, agencies which employ these mental health professionals include the Department of Defense, the Veterans Health Administration (within the Department of Veterans Affairs), the Bureau of Prisons (within the Department of Justice), and the Indian Health Service (within HHS), among other agencies. The federal government is the largest employer of some provider types, such as clinical psychologists and social workers. [24] As such, the cost of employing different provider types—as well as their scopes of practice—may be a consideration not only in determining staffing priorities, but also in attempts to recruit and retain mental health providers (e.g., by offering competitive compensation).

## APPENDIX A. MENTAL HEALTH PROFESSIONAL SHORTAGE AREAS (MHPSA) DEFINITION

This appendix excerpts the specific criteria that the Health Resources and Services Administration (HRSA) uses to designate mental health professional shortage areas (MHPSAs). MHPSAs can be geographic areas, population groups, or facilities. This designation is used to determine eligibility for federal programs such as Medicare bonus payments and health professions recruitment programs.[25] HRSA bases the MHPSA designation on the availability (relative to population size) of "core mental health professionals," which include "psychiatrists, clinical psychologists, clinical social workers, psychiatric nurse specialists, and marriage and family therapists." The criteria for designating a MHPSA are as follows:[26]

1. Geographic Areas must:
- Be a rational area for the delivery of mental health services
- Meet one of the following conditions:
  - A population-to-core-mental-health-professional ratio greater than or equal to 6,000:1 and a population-to-psychiatrist ratio greater than or equal to 20,000:1 or
  - A population-to-core professional ratio greater than or equal to 9,000:1 or
  - A population-to-psychiatrist ratio greater than or equal to 30,000:1
- Have unusually high needs for mental health services, and
  - A population-to-core-mental-health-professional ratio greater than or equal to 4,500:1 and a population-to-psychiatrist ratio greater than or equal to 15,000:1, or
  - A population-to-core-professional ratio greater than or equal to 6,000:1, or
  - A population-to-psychiatrist ratio greater than or equal to 20,000:1
- Mental health professionals in contiguous areas are overutilized, excessively distant or inaccessible to residents of the area under consideration.

2. Population Groups must:
- Face access barriers that prevent the population group from use of the area's mental health providers
- Meet one of the following criteria:
  - Have a ratio of the number of persons in the population group to the number of FTE core mental health professionals serving the population group greater than or equal to 4,500:1 and the ratio of the number of persons in the population group to the number of FTE psychiatrists serving the population group greater than or equal to 15,000:1; or
  - Have a ratio of the number of persons in the population group to the number of FTE core mental health professionals serving the population group greater than or equal to 6,000:1; or

- o Have a ratio of the number of persons in the population group to the number of FTE psychiatrists serving the population group are greater than or equal to 20,000:1

3. Facilities must:
- Be maximum or medium security facilities
- Be either Federal and/or State correctional institutions, State/County mental hospitals or public and/or non-profit mental health facilities
- Federal or State Correctional facilities must:
  - o Have at least 250 inmates and
  - o Have a ratio of the number of internees per year to the number of FTE [full-time equivalent] psychiatrists serving the institution of at least 2,000:1
- State and county mental health hospitals must:
  - o Have an average daily inpatient amount of at least 100; and
  - o The number of workload units per FTE psychiatrists available at the hospital exceeds 300, where workload units are calculated using the following formula: Total workload units = average daily inpatient census + 2 x (number of inpatient admissions per year) + 0.5 x (number of admissions to day care and outpatient services per year).
- Community mental health centers and other public and non-profit facilities must:
  - o Be providing (or responsible for providing) mental health services to an area or population group designated as having a shortage of mental health professionals and
  - o Have insufficient capacity to meet the psychiatric needs of the area or population group

B. *Methodology.*[27]

*In determining whether an area meets the criteria... the following methodology will be used:*

1. *Rational Areas for the Delivery of Mental Health Services.*
   *(a) The following areas will be considered rational areas for the delivery of mental health services:*

i. An established mental health catchment area, as designated in the State Mental Health Plan under the general criteria set forth in section 238 of the Community Mental Health Centers Act.
ii. A portion of an established mental health catchment area whose population, because of topography, market and/or transportation patterns or other factors, has limited access to mental health resources in the rest of the catchment area, as measured generally by a travel time of greater than 40 minutes to these resources.
iii. A county or metropolitan area which contains more than one mental health catchment area, where data are unavailable by individual catchment area.

(b) *The following distances will be used as guidelines in determining distances corresponding to 40 minutes travel time:*
i. Under normal conditions with primary roads available: 25 miles.
ii. In mountainous terrain or in areas with only secondary roads available: 20 miles.
iii. In flat terrain or in areas connected by interstate highways: 30 miles.

Within inner portions of metropolitan areas, information on the public transportation system will be used to determine the distance corresponding to 40 minutes travel time.

2. *Population Count.*

The population count used will be the total permanent resident civilian population of the area, excluding inmates of institutions.

3. *Counting of mental health professionals.*

(a) All non-Federal core mental health professionals (as defined below) providing mental health patient care (direct or other, including consultation and supervision) in ambulatory or other short-term care settings to residents of the area will be counted. Data on each type of core professional should be presented separately, in terms of the number of full-time-equivalent (FTE) practitioners of each type represented.

(b) *Definitions:*
i. Core mental health professionals or core professionals includes those psychiatrists, clinical psychologists, clinical social

workers, psychiatric nurse specialists, and marriage and family therapists who meet the definitions below.

ii. Psychiatrist means a doctor of medicine (M.D.) or doctor of osteopathy (D.O.) who

*(A) Is certified as a psychiatrist or child psychiatrist by the American Medical Specialties Board of Psychiatry and Neurology or by the American Osteopathic Board of Neurology and Psychiatry, or, if not certified, is "board-eligible" (i.e., has successfully completed an accredited program of graduate medical or osteopathic education in psychiatry or child psychiatry); and*

*(B) Practices patient care psychiatry or child psychiatry, and is licensed to do so, if required by the State of practice.*

iii. Clinical psychologist means an individual (normally with a doctorate in psychology) who is practicing as a clinical or counseling psychologist and is licensed or certified to do so by the State of practice; or, if licensure or certification is not required in the State of practice, an individual with a doctorate in psychology and two years of supervised clinical or counseling experience. (School psychologists are not included.)

*Clinical social worker means an individual who—*

*(A) Is certified as a clinical social worker by the American Board of Examiners in Clinical Social Work, or is listed on the National Association of Social Workers' Clinical Register, or has a master's degree in social work and two years of supervised clinical experience; and*

*(B) Is licensed to practice as a social worker, if required by the State of practice.*

iv. Psychiatric nurse specialist means a registered nurse (R.N.) who—

*(A) Is certified by the American Nurses Association as a psychiatric and mental health clinical nurse specialist, or has a master's degree in nursing with a specialization in psychiatric/mental health and two years of supervised clinical experience; and*

*(B) Is licensed to practice as a psychiatric or mental health nurse specialist, if required by the State of practice.*

v. Marriage and family therapist means an individual (normally with a master's or doctoral degree in marital and family therapy and at least two years of supervised clinical experience) who is practicing as a marital and family therapist and is licensed or certified to do so by the State of practice; or, if licensure or certification is not required by the State of practice, is eligible for clinical membership in the American Association for Marriage and Family Therapy.

## APPENDIX B. ADDITIONAL RESOURCES

Below are resources for additional information about each mental health provider type, including national associations of state boards, professional associations, accrediting organizations for educational programs, and other relevant organizations. In some cases, a single organization may serve multiple roles (e.g., a professional association may also accredit educational programs).

### Psychiatrists

American Academy of Addiction Psychiatry (AAAP): http://www2.aaap.org
American Academy of Child & Adolescent Psychiatry (AACAP): http://www.aacap.org
American Academy of Clinical Psychiatrists (AACP): https://www.aacp.com
American Board of Medical Specialties (ABMS): http://www.abms.org
American Board of Psychiatry and Neurology (ABPN): http://www.abpn.com
American Psychiatric Association (APA): http://www.psych.org
National Board of Osteopathic Examiners: http://www.nbome.org

### Psychologists

American Psychological Association (APA): http://www.apa.org
Association of State and Provincial Psychology Boards (ASPPB):http://www.asppb.net

### Social Workers

Association of Social Work Boards (ASWB): http://www.aswb.org

Council on Social Work Education (CSWE): http://www.cswe.org
National Association of Social Workers (NASW): http://www.socialworkers.org
Social Work Policy Institute (SWPI): http://www.socialworkpolicy.org

## Advanced Practice Psychiatric Nurses

American Academy of Nurse Practitioners (AANP): http://www.aanp.org
American Nurses Credentialing Center (ANCC): http://www.nursecredentialing.org
American Psychiatric Nurses Association (APNA): http://www.apna.org
National Association of Clinical Nurse Specialists (NACNS): http://www.nacns.org National Council of State Boards of Nursing (NCSBN): https://www.ncsbn.org

## Marriage and Family Therapists

American Association for Marriage and Family Therapy (AAMFT): http://www.aamft.org
Association of Marital and Family Therapy Regulatory Boards (AMFTRB): http://www.amftrb.org

## End Notes

[1] For example, federal agencies such as the Veterans Health Administration (within the Department of Veterans Affairs) provide mental health care directly; federal programs such as Medicare pay for mental health care; and federal agencies such as the Substance Abuse and Mental Health Services Administration (within the Department of Health and Human Services) support mental health care through grant funding, dissemination of best practices, technical assistance, and other means.

[2] See, for example, U.S. Congress, Senate Committee on Health, Education, Labor, and Pensions, Assessing the State of America's Mental Health System, 113th Cong., 1st sess., January 24, 2013; U.S. Congress, House Committee on Veterans' Affairs, Honoring the Commitment: Overcoming Barriers to Quality Mental Health Care for Veterans, 113th Cong., 1st sess., February 13, 2013; U.S. Congress, Senate Committee on Veterans' Affairs, VA Mental Health Care: Ensuring Timely Access to High-Quality Care, 113th Cong., 1st sess., March 20, 2013; and U.S. Congress, House Energy & Commerce Committee, Oversight and Investigations Subcommittee, Examining SAMHSA's Role in Delivering Services to the

Severely Mentally Ill, 113th Cong., 1st sess., May 22, 2013. (SAMHSA is the abbreviation for the Substance Abuse and Mental Health Services Administration.)

[3] For example, in the 113th Congress, bills have been introduced intended to improve mental health care overall (e.g., H.R. 1263, S. 264, and S. 689), and for specific populations such as veterans (e.g., H.R. 1725 and H.R. 2540), school children (e.g., H.R. 320 and H.R. 628), and Medicare beneficiaries (e.g., H.R. 794 and S. 562), among others.

[4] IOM (Institute of Medicine). 2012. The Mental Health and Substance Use Workforce for Older Adults: In Whose Hands? Washington, DC: The National Academies Press. Hereinafter, IOM Workforce Report. The IOM definition also includes all fields in the SAMHSA definitions.

[5] SAMHSA. (2012). Mental Health, United States, 2010. HHS Publication No. (SMA) 12-4681. Rockville, MD: SAMHSA.

[6] Substance Abuse and Mental Health Services Administration (SAMHSA). (2006) Mental Health, United States, 2004. HHS Publication No. (SMA) 06-4195. Rockville, MD: SAMHSA. The IOM definition includes all fields in the SAMHSA definitions.

[7] HRSA, About HRSA, http://www.hrsa.gov/about/.

[8] Health professions shortage areas (HPSAs) are defined in 42 U.S.C. §254e. HRSA developed operational definitions of HPSAs and of MHPSAs specifically, available at http://bhpr.hrsa.gov/shortage/hpsas/designationcriteria/ designationcriteria.html and http://bhpr.hrsa.gov/shortage/hpsas/designationcriteria/mentalhealthhpsaoverview.html. HRSA designates MHPSAs based on the ratio of mental health providers to population. As of June 2013, HRSA had designated 3,744 MHPSAs. See U.S. Department of Health and Human Services, Health Resources and Services Administration, "Health Professional Shortage Areas (HPSA) and Medically Underserved Areas/Populations (MUA/P)," http://datawarehouse.hrsa.gov/hpsadetail.aspx. For a larger discussion of Health Professional Shortage Areas (HPSAs, of which MHPSAs are a specific type), see CRS Report R42029, Physician Supply and the Affordable Care Act, by Elayne J. Heisler.

[9] This report uses the term "advanced practice psychiatric nurse," which is more common than the term "psychiatric nurse specialists" used in HRSA's MHPSA designation criteria. See U.S. Department of Health and Human Services, Health Resources and Services Administration, "Mental Health HPSA Designation Overview," http://bhpr.hrsa.gov/shortage/hpsas/designationcriteria/mentalhealthhpsaoverview.html.

[10] The HRSA definition is used because of its relevance to federal workforce programs.

[11] See, for example, "FSMB Mission and Goals," Federation of State Medical Boards at http://www.fsmb.org/ mission.html.

[12] In order for a health professional to "count" for MHPSA designation purposes, the health professional must be licensed to practice independently.

[13] As licensure requirements change over time, previously licensed providers may not be subject to new requirements.

[14] Some disciplines offer degrees with the same title in both clinical and non-clinical tracks—for example, a Doctor of Philosophy (PhD) in clinical psychology and a PhD in experimental psychology or a Masters of Social Work (MSW) in clinical social work and an MSW social work administration—where graduates of the non-clinical track are not qualified for clinical licensure.

[15] Licensure generally requires a degree from a school or program that has been accredited; however, a discussion of accreditation of educational institutions and programs is beyond the scope of this report.

[16] One of the primary challenges in assessing the overall size of the mental health workforce is that there is no uniform definition; see "Mental Health Workforce Definition." Using the HRSA definition of "core mental health professionals," a relatively narrow definition, yields a smaller estimate than would be found using a somewhat broader definition such as the one used by SAMSHA or a much broader definition such as the one used by the IOM.

[17] Health Resources and Services Administration, Data Warehouse, Health Professional Shortage Areas (HPSA) and Medically Underserved Areas / Populations (MUA/P), http://datawarehouse.hrsa.gov/hpsadetail.aspx.

[18] HRSA uses a variety of data sources when designating MHPSAs. Individual states apply to HRSA for MHPSA designations. When doing so states must provide data on the ratio of health practitioners to population. States use a variety of sources when providing these data including professional association data, state licensing data, and state specific survey data. Source: E-mail from HHS Office of the Assistant Secretary for Legislation, August 1, 2013.

[19] Institute of Medicine. (2012). The Mental Health and Substance Use Workforce for Older Adults: In Whose Hands? Washington, DC: The National Academies Press. IOM is a private, nonprofit institution established in 1970 under the congressional charter of the National Academy of Sciences to provide health policy advice. See National Academies, Institute of Medicine, About the IOM, http://www.iom.edu/About-IOM.aspx. For information about the health professions included in the IOM's definition of the mental health workforce, see "Mental Health Workforce Definition."

[20] Substance Abuse and Mental Health Services Administration (SAMHSA). (2012). Mental Health, United States, 2010. HHS Publication No. (SMA) 12-4681. Rockville, MD: SAMHSA. SAMHSA is a public health agency established within HHS by Congress in 1992 to advance mental health in the United States. See SAMHSA, About Us, http://beta.samhsa.gov/about-us. For information about the health professions included in the SAMSHA's definition of the mental health workforce, see "Mental Health Workforce Definition: No Consensus."

[21] For example, the BLS Handbook of Methods, Chapter 3: Occupational Employment Statistics discusses the uses of the OES data that include federal programs, state workforce agencies, and the Department of Labor Foreign Labor Certification Program, see http://www.bls.gov/opub/hom/homch3.htm#uses.

[22] CRS Report R42029, Physician Supply and the Affordable Care Act, by Elayne J. Heisler, discusses the interplay between the demand for health services and the supply of a specific type of providers: physicians. Some of the discussion and some of the policy levers used to affect physician supply could also be used to affect the mental health workforce. For a description of health workforce programs, see CRS Report R41278, Public Health, Workforce, Quality, and Related Provisions in ACA: Summary and Timeline, coordinated by C. Stephen Redhead and Elayne J. Heisler; CRS Report R42029, Physician Supply and the Affordable Care Act, by Elayne J. Heisler; and U.S. Government Accountability Office (GAO), Health Care Workforce: Federally Funded Training Programs in Fiscal Year 2012, 13-709R, August 15, 2013, http://www.gao.gov/products/GAO-13-709R.

[23] BLS projects the growth rate between 2010 and 2020 to be 14% among all occupations, 26% among health care practitioners, and higher within some of the mental health professions (e.g., 41% among marriage and family therapists and 31% among mental health and substance abuse social workers). Department of Labor, Bureau of Labor Statistics, "Employment Projections, Employment by Occupation," February 1, 2012, http://www.bls.gov/emp/ep_table_102.htm.

[24] See, for example, U.S. Congress, House Committee on Veterans' Affairs, Subcommittee on Health, Human Resources Challenges with the Veterans Health Administration, committee print, prepared by Randy Phelps, Deputy Executive Director for Professional Practice of the American Psychological Association, 110th Cong., May 22, 2008, http://veterans.house.gov/witness-testimony/randy-phelps-phd; psychologist recruiting information from the Federal Bureau of Prisons at http://www.bop.gov/jobs/hsd/ psychology_services.jspl; and social work recruiting information from the Department of Veterans Affairs at http://www.vacareers.va.gov/resources/downloads/MHEI_Brochure.pdf.

In: U.S. Mental Health Workforce ...
Editor: Maurice Gordon

ISBN: 978-1-62948-865-3
© 2014 Nova Science Publishers, Inc.

*Chapter 2*

# STATEMENT OF PAMELA S. HYDE, ADMINISTRATOR, SUBSTANCE ABUSE AND MENTAL HEALTH SERVICES ADMINISTRATION. HEARING ON "ASSESSING THE STATE OF AMERICA'S MENTAL HEALTH SYSTEM"[*]

Chairman Harkin, Ranking Member Alexander and members of the Senate Health, Education, Labor, and Pensions Committee, thank you for inviting me to testify at this important hearing on the state of the mental health system. I am pleased to testify along with Dr. Insel on the state of America's mental health system and to discuss some of the initiatives related to mental health included in the President's plan to protect our children and our communities.

## THE SUBSTANCE ABUSE AND MENTAL HEALTH SERVICES ADMINISTRATION (SAMHSA)

As you are aware, the Substance Abuse and Mental Health Services Administration's (SAMHSA) mission is to reduce the impact of substance

---

[*] This is an edited, reformatted and augmented version of a statement presented January 24, 2013 before the Senate Committee on Health, Education, Labor, and Pensions.

abuse and mental illness on America's communities. SAMHSA envisions a Nation that acts on the knowledge that:

- Behavioral health is essential for health;
- Prevention works;
- Treatment is effective; and
- People recover from mental and substance use disorders.

In order to achieve this mission, SAMHSA has identified eight Strategic Initiatives to focus the Agency's work on improving lives and capitalizing on emerging opportunities. SAMHSA's top Strategic Initiatives are: Prevention; Trauma and Justice; Health Reform; Military Families; Recovery Supports; Health Information Technology; Data, Outcomes and Quality; and Public Awareness and Support.

## PREVALENCE OF BEHAVIORAL HEALTH CONDITIONS AND TREATMENT

In the wake of the Newtown tragedy, it is important to note that behavioral health research and practice over the last 20 years reveal that most people who are violent do not have a mental disorder, and most people with a mental disorder are not violent.[1] Studies indicate that people with mental illnesses are more likely to be the victims of violent attacks than the general population.[2] In fact, demographic variables such as age, gender and socioeconomic status are more reliable predictors of violence than mental illness.[3] These facts are important because misconceptions about mental illness can cause discrimination and unfairly hamper the recovery of the nearly 20 percent of all adult Americans who experience a mental illness each year.

It is estimated that almost half of all Americans will experience symptoms of a mental health condition – mental illness or addiction – at some point in their lives. Yet, today, less than one in five children and adolescents with diagnosable mental health problems receive the treatment they need.[4] And according to data from SAMHSA's National Survey on Drug Use and Health (NSDUH), only 38% of adults with diagnosable mental health problems – and only 11% of those with diagnosable substance use disorders - receive needed treatment.[5]

With respect to the onset of behavioral health conditions, half of all lifetime cases of mental and substance use disorders begin by age 14 and three-fourths by age 24.[6] When persons with mental health conditions or substance use disorders do not receive the proper treatment and supportive services they need, crisis situations can arise affecting individuals, families, schools, and communities. We need to do more to identify mental health and substance abuse issues early and help individuals get the treatment they need before these crisis situations develop. And we need to help communities understand and implement the prevention approaches we know can be effective in stopping issues from developing in the first place.

The President's announcement includes several important steps to help address mental health prevention and treatment. I look forward to the opportunity to discuss these with you.

## MENTAL HEALTH FINANCING

First, however, I will provide some background on mental health financing. The National Expenditures for Mental Health Services and Substance Abuse Treatment report for 1986-2005 found that $113 billion was spent on mental health and $22 billion for substance abuse services in 2005. SAMHSA is in the process of updating this data. In 2005, spending on mental health services accounted for 6.1 percent of all-health spending. Public payers accounted for 58 percent of mental health spending and 46 percent of all-health spending. Medicaid (28 percent of mental health spending) and private insurance (27 percent of mental health spending) accounted for more than half of mental health spending in 2005, followed by other State and local government at 18 percent, Medicare at 8 percent, out-of-pocket at 12 percent, other Federal at 5 percent and other private sources at 3 percent.

The National Expenditures report also found prescription drugs accounted for the largest share of mental health spending in 2005—27 percent. Mental health drug spending grew by an average of 24 percent a year between 1997 and 2001. After 2001, growth slowed dramatically, to an average rate of 10 percent a year between 2001 and 2005.

A key source of funding for services for adults with serious mental illness (SMI) and children with severe emotional disturbances (SED) is the Community Mental Health Services Block Grant (MHBG), which is a flexible funding source that is used by States to provide a range of mental health services described in their plans for comprehensive community-based mental health services for children with serious emotional disturbance and adults with serious mental illness. These funds are used to support service delivery through planning, administration, evaluation, educational activities, and services. Services include rehabilitation services, crisis stabilization and case management, peer specialist and consumer-directed services, wrap around services for children and families, supported employment and housing, jail diversion programs, and services for special populations. The State plan is developed in collaboration with the State mental health planning councils. Planning Councils' membership is statutorily mandated to include consumers, family members of adult and child consumers, providers, and representatives of other principal State agencies. The FY 2013 President's Budget proposed $460 million to continue the MHBG.

SAMHSA also administers the Substance Abuse Prevention and Treatment Block Grant (SABG) for the States. The FY 2013 President's Budget proposed $1.4 billion for the SABG, and $400 million for primary prevention of substance abuse.

According to the National Association of State Mental Health Program Directors, over the past few years, States and communities have significantly reduced funding for mental health and addiction services. They estimate that in the last four years, States have cut $4.35 billion in mental health services, while an additional 700,000 people sought help at public mental health facilities during this period.[7]

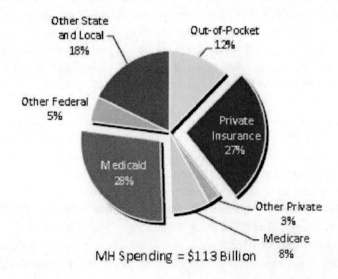

Distribution of Spending on MH Treatment by Payer, 2005

MH Spending = $113 Billion

These changes have occurred despite the evidence that early treatment and prevention for mental illness and substance use programs can reduce health costs, criminal and juvenile justice costs, and educational costs, and increase productivity.[8]

Additionally, investments in these programs and services can help reduce physical health costs for those with co-morbid health and behavioral health conditions.[9] Some States have found that providing adequate mental health and addiction-treatment benefits can dramatically reduce health care costs and Medicaid spending.

## ADVANCEMENTS AND TRENDS IN BEHAVIORAL HEALTH

### Community-Based Care

In 1963, President John F. Kennedy signed into law the Mental Retardation Facilities and Community Mental Health Centers Construction Act. The Act led to a drastic alteration in the delivery of mental health services and establishment of more than 750 comprehensive community mental health centers throughout the country. This movement to community-based services helped to reduce the number of individuals with mental illness who were "warehoused" in secluded hospitals and isolated institutions. Other advancements in the treatment of mental illness and the growth of the recovery movement, along with other programs such as supportive housing, assertive community treatment teams, peer specialists, supportive employment, and social security disability payments, have helped provide the services and supports necessary for persons with serious mental illness to survive and thrive in the community. Experience and research has shown that the goal of recovery is exemplified through a life that includes: Health; Home; Purpose and Community.[10]

Peers play an important role in recovery support and the consumer movement has helped promote not only the idea that recovery is possible, but also those consumers should play a key role in their recovery. SAMHSA's Recovery Support Initiative partners with people in recovery from mental and substance use disorders and family members to guide the behavioral health system and promote individual-, program-, and system-level approaches that foster health and resilience; increase permanent housing, employment, education, and other necessary supports; and reduce discriminatory barriers.

## Integration

Given that behavioral health is essential to an individual's overall health, SAMHSA administers the Primary and Behavioral Health Care Integration (PBHCI) program. The purpose of the program is to improve the physical health status of people with serious mental illnesses (SMI) by supporting communities to coordinate and integrate primary care services into publicly funded community mental health and other community-based behavioral health settings.

The program supports community-based behavioral health agencies' efforts to build the partnerships and infrastructure needed to initiate or expand the provision of primary healthcare services for people in treatment for SMI and co-occurring SMI and substance use disorders. It is a program focused on increasing the health status of individuals based on physical or behavioral need. The program encourages structural changes in existing systems to accomplish its goals.

To date, the program has awarded 94 grants and 55 percent of awardees are partnering with at least one Federally Qualified Health Center (FQHC). This integration results in significant physical and behavioral health gains. PBHCI grantees collect data on patients at admission and in follow-up reassessments every six months, as well as at discharge when possible. Some results that are based on grantee-reported outcome measures from February 2010 through January 7, 2013, include:

- Health: The percentage of consumers who rated their overall health as positive increased by 20% from baseline to most recent reassessment (N=3737).
- Tobacco Use: The percentage of consumers who reported they were not using tobacco during the past 30 days increased by 6% from baseline to most recent reassessment (N=3787).
- Illegal Substance Use: The percentage of consumers who reported that they were not using an illegal substance during the past 30 days increased by 12% from baseline to most recent reassessment (N=3568).

- Blood pressure (categorical): Among 7493 clients, 18.3% showed improvement, and 16.7% are no longer at risk for high blood pressure (systolic less than 130, diastolic less than 85).
- BMI: Among 7120 clients, 45.6% showed improvement, and 4.8% are no longer at risk for being overweight (BMI less than 25).

Service systems that are aligned with patient and client need, specifically those providing integrated treatment, produce better outcomes for individuals with co-occurring mental and substance use disorders.[11]

Without integrated treatment, one or both disorders may not be addressed properly. Mental health and substance abuse authorities across the country are taking steps to integrate systems and services, and promote integrated behavioral health treatment. Currently, there are thirty-five States that have a combined mental health and substance abuse authority. In addition, at least two additional States and the District of Columbia are moving toward a single agency.

SAMHSA continues to work with both States and grantees to encourage systems collaboration and coordination to develop mental health and substance abuse systems that support seamless service delivery. SAMHSA's effort to integrate primary care and mental health and substance abuse services offers a promising, viable, and efficient way of ensuring that people have access to needed behavioral health services. Additionally, behavioral health care delivered in a primary care setting can help to minimize discrimination and reduce negative attitude about seeking services, while increasing opportunities to improve overall health outcomes. Leadership supporting this type of coordinated quality care requires the support of a strengthened behavioral health and primary care delivery system as well as a long-term policy commitment.

## Mental Health Parity and Addiction Equity Act (MHPAEA)

In 2008, the Paul Wellstone and Pete Domenici Mental Health Parity and Addiction Equity Act (MHPAEA) became law. MHPAEA improves access to much needed mental and substance use disorder treatment services through more equitable coverage. The law applied to large group health plans (sponsored by employers with more than 50 employees) and health insurance issuers that offered coverage in the large group market. The law requires that plans and issuers that offer coverage for mental illness and substance use disorders provide those benefits in a way that is no more restrictive than the predominant requirements or limitations applied to substantially all medical and surgical benefits covered by the plan.

## Affordable Care Act

The Affordable Care Act advances the field of behavioral health by expanding access to behavioral health care; growing the country's behavioral health workforce; reducing behavioral health disparities; and implementing the science of behavioral health promotion. While most mental illnesses and addictions are treatable, those with mental illness often cannot get needed treatment if they do not have health insurance that covers mental health services. The Affordable Care Act will provide one of the largest expansions of mental health and substance abuse coverage in a generation by extending health coverage to over 30 million Americans, including an estimated 6 to 10 million people with mental illness. It also includes coverage for preventive services, including screening for depression and alcohol misuse. The Affordable Care Act will also make sure that Americans can get the mental health treatment they need by ensuring that insurance plans in the new Marketplaces cover mental health and substance abuse benefits at parity with other benefits. Beginning in 2014, all new small group and individual plans will cover mental health and substance use disorder services, including behavioral health treatment. Medicaid is already the largest payer of mental health services, and the Affordable Care Act will extend Medicaid coverage to as many as 17 million hardworking Americans.

SAMHSA's number one strategic initiative is Prevention of Substance Abuse and Mental Illness, and the Agency has also been heavily engaged in the implementation of the prevention and public health promotion provisions of the Affordable Care Act. For example, the National Prevention Strategy includes priorities focused on Mental and Emotional Well-Being and Preventing Drug Abuse and Excessive Alcohol Use.

## MOVING FORWARD

Moving forward, in the wake of the tragedy in Newtown, CT, the Administration is focused on making sure that students and young adults get treatment for mental health issues. At the same time, SAMHSA knows that a larger national dialogue about mental health in America needs to occur and we will be taking steps to foster this dialogue.

## Parity

The Administration intends to issue next month the Final Rule on defining essential health benefits and implementing requirements for new small group and individual plans to cover mental health benefits at parity with medical and surgical benefits. In addition, the President announced that the Administration is committed to promulgating a MHPAEA Final Rule.

Last week, the Centers for Medicare and Medicaid Services sent a State Health Official Letter regarding the applicability of MHPAEA to Medicaid non-managed care benchmark and benchmark-equivalent plans (referred to in this letter as Medicaid Alternative Benefit plans) as described in section 1937 of the Social Security Act (the Act), the Children's Health Insurance Programs (CHIP) under title XXI of the Act, and Medicaid managed care programs as described in section 1932 of the Act.

## Reaching Youth and Young Adults

As I noted earlier, three-quarters of mental illnesses appear by the age of 24, yet less than one in five children and adolescents with diagnosable mental health and substance use problems receive treatment. That is why last week, the President announced initiatives to ensure that students and young adults receive treatment for mental health issues. Specifically, SAMHSA will take a leadership role in initiatives that would:

- Reach 750,000 young people through programs to identify mental illness early and refer them to treatment: We need to train teachers and other adults who regularly interact with students to recognize young people who need help and ensure they are referred to mental health services. The Administration is calling for a new initiative, Project AWARE (Advancing Wellness and Resilience in Education), to provide this training and set up systems to provide these referrals. This initiative has two parts:
  o Provide "Mental Health First Aid" training for teachers: Project AWARE proposes $15 million for training for teachers and other

adults who interact with youth to detect and respond to mental illness in children and young adults, including how to encourage adolescents and families experiencing these problems to seek treatment.
  - Make sure students with signs of mental illness get referred to treatment: Project AWARE also proposes $40 million to help school districts work with law enforcement, mental health agencies, and other local organizations to assure students with mental health issues or other behavioral issues are referred to and receive the services they need. This initiative builds on strategies that, for over a decade, have proven to improve mental health.
- Support individuals ages 16 to 25 at high risk for mental illness: Efforts to help youth and young adults cannot end when a student leaves high school. Individuals ages 16 to 25 are at high risk for mental illness, substance abuse, and suicide, but they are among the least likely to seek help. Even those who received services as a child may fall through the cracks when they turn 18. The Administration is proposing $25 million for innovative State-based strategies supporting young people ages 16 to 25 with mental health or substance abuse issues.
- Train more than 5,000 additional mental health professionals to serve students and young adults: Experts often cite the shortage of mental health service providers as one reason it can be hard to access treatment. To help fill this gap, the Administration is proposing $50 million to train social workers, counselors, psychologists, and other mental health professionals. This would provide stipends and tuition reimbursement to train more than 5,000 mental health professionals serving young people in our schools and communities.

## National Dialogue

Finally, we know that it is time to change the conversation about mental illness and mental health in America. HHS is working to develop a national dialogue on the mental and emotional health of our young people, engaging parents, peers, and teachers to reduce negative attitudes toward people with mental illness, to recognize the warning signs, and to enhance access to treatment.

## CONCLUSION

Thank you again for this opportunity to discuss the state of America's mental health system. I would be pleased to answer any questions that you may have.

## End Notes

[1] Monahan J, Steadman H, Silver E, et al: Rethinking Risk Assessment: The MacArthur Study of Mental Disorder and Violence. New York, Oxford University Press, 2001 and Swanson, 1994.

[2] Appleby, L., Mortensen, P. B., Dunn, G., & Hiroeh, U. (2001). Death by homicide, suicide, and other unnatural causes in people with mental illness: a population-based study. The Lancet, 358, 2110-2112.

[3] Elbogen EB, Johnson SC. Arch Gen Psychiatry. 2009 Feb;66(2):152-61. doi: 10.1001/archgenpsychiatry.2008.537. The intricate link between violence and mental disorder: results from the National Epidemiologic Survey on Alcohol and Related Conditions.

[4] Unmet Need for Mental Health Care Among U.S. Children: Variation by Ethnicity and Insurance Status Sheryl H. Kataoka, M.D., M.S.H.S.; Lily Zhang, M.S.; Kenneth B. Wells, M.D., M.P.H., Am J Psychiatry 2002;159:1548-1555. 10.1176/appi.ajp.159.9.1548

[5] Substance Abuse and Mental Health Services Administration, Results from the 2011 National Survey on Drug Use and Health: Mental Health Findings, NSDUH Series H-45, HHS Publication No. (SMA) 12-4725. Rockville, MD: Substance Abuse and Mental Health Services Administration, 2012.

[6] Kessler, R. C., Berglund, P., Demler, O., Jin, R., Merikangas, K. R., & Walters, E. E. (2005). Lifetime prevalence and age-of-onset distributions of DSMIV disorders in the National Comorbidity Survey Replication. Archives of General Psychiatry, 62(6), 593–602.

[7] The National Association of State Mental Health Program Directors (NASMHPD). Too Significant To Fail: The Importance of State Behavioral Health Agencies in the Daily Lives of Americans with Mental Illness, for Their Families, and for Their Communities. Alexandria, VA. 2012.

[8] National Research Council. Preventing Mental, Emotional, and Behavioral Disorders Among Young People: Progress and Possibilities. Washington, DC: The National Academies Press, 2009.

[9] See e.g., Egede, L.E., Zheng, D., & Simpson, K. (2002). Comorbid depression is associated with increased health care use and expenditures in individuals with diabetes. Diabetes Care, 25(3), 464-470.

[10] New Freedom Commission on Mental Health, Achieving the Promise: Transforming Mental Health Care in America. Final Report. DHHS Pub. No. SMA-03-3832. Rockville, MD: 2003.

[11] Center for Substance Abuse Treatment. Systems Integration. COCE Overview Paper 7. DHHS Publication No. (SMA) 07-4295. Rockville, MD: Substance Abuse and Mental Health Services Administration, and Center for Mental Health Services, 2007.

*Chapter 3*

# TESTIMONY OF THOMAS INSEL, DIRECTOR, NATIONAL INSTITUTE OF MENTAL HEALTH. HEARING ON "ASSESSING THE STATE OF AMERICA'S MENTAL HEALTH SYSTEM"[*]

Mr. Chairman and Members of the Committee:

I am Thomas R. Insel, M.D., Director of the National Institute of Mental Health (NIMH) at the National Institutes of Health, an agency in the Department of Health and Human Services. Thank you for this opportunity to present an overview of the current state of mental health research at NIMH, with a particular focus on our efforts to address serious mental illness, and our efforts to discover, develop, and pursue new treatments for these brain disorders. In my statement, I will review the scope of mental disorders in the United States and their impact on public health, and I will outline examples of NIMH's research efforts designed to address this challenge.

## PUBLIC HEALTH BURDEN OF MENTAL ILLNESS

The National Institute of Mental Health is the lead Federal agency for research on mental disorders, with a mission to transform the understanding and treatment of mental illnesses through basic and clinical research. The

---

[*] This is an edited, reformatted and augmented version of a Testimony, Presented January 24, 2013 before the Senate Committee on Health, Education, Labor, and Pensions.

burden of mental illness is enormous. In the United States, an estimated 11.4 million American adults (approximately 4.4 percent of all adults) suffer from a serious mental illness (SMI) each year, including conditions such as schizophrenia, bipolar disorder, and major depression.[1] According to a 2004 World Health Organization report, neuropsychiatric disorders are the leading cause of disability in the United States and Canada, accounting for 28 percent of all years of life lost to disability and premature mortality (Disability Adjusted Life Years or DALYs).[2] The personal, social and economic costs associated with these disorders are tremendous. Suicide is the 10th leading cause of death in the United States, accounting for the loss of more than 38,000 American lives each year, more than double the number of lives lost to homicide.[3] A cautious estimate places the direct and indirect financial costs associated with mental illness in the United States at well over $300 billion annually, and it ranks as the third most costly medical condition in terms of overall health care expenditure, behind only heart conditions and traumatic injury.[4,5] Even more concerning, the burden of illness for mental disorders is projected to sharply increase, not decrease, over the next 20 years.[6]

NIMH-supported research has found that Americans with SMI die eight years earlier than the general population.[7] People with SMI experience chronic medical conditions and the risk factors that contribute to them more frequently and at earlier ages. There are low rates of prevention, detection, and intervention for chronic medical conditions and their risk factors among people with SMI, and this contributes to significant illness and earlier death. Two-thirds or more of adults with SMI smoke[8]; over 40 percent are obese (60 percent for women)[9,10]; and metabolic syndrome is highly prevalent, especially in women.[11] Approximately five percent of individuals with schizophrenia will die by suicide during their lifetime, a rate 50-fold greater than the general population.[12]

## DELAYS IN RECEIVING TREATMENT— AND THE CONSEQUENCES

According to a study published in 2004, the vast majority (80.1 percent) of people having any mental disorder eventually make contact with a health care professional to receive treatment, although delays to seeking care average more than a decade.[13] Although instances of SMI are associated with shorter delays, the average delay was nevertheless approximately five years— that is five years of increased risk for using potentially life-threatening, self-administered treatments, such as legal or illicit substances, or even death. During an episode of psychosis, people can lose touch with reality and experience hallucinations and delusions. Research has suggested that persons with schizophrenia whose psychotic symptoms are controlled are no more violent than those without SMI.[14] Nonetheless, when untreated psychosis is also accompanied by symptoms of paranoia and when it is associated with substance abuse, the risk of violence is increased. Importantly, the risk of violence is reduced with appropriate treatment. Moreover, people with SMI are 11 times more likely than the general population to be victims themselves of violence.[15]

## HOW NIMH IS ADDRESSING THIS PUBLIC HEALTH CHALLENGE

In the past, we viewed mental disorders as chronic conditions defined by their apparent symptoms, even though behavioral manifestations of illness are in fact the last indications— following a cascade of subtle brain changes—that something is wrong. We understand now that mental disorders are brain disorders, with specific symptoms rooted in abnormal patterns of brain activity. Moving forward, NIMH aims to support research on earlier diagnosis and quicker delivery of appropriate treatment, be it behavioral or pharmacological. NIMH has a three-pronged research approach to achieve this aim: (1) optimize early treatment to improve the trajectory of illness in people who are already experiencing the symptoms of SMI; (2) understand and prevent the transition from the pre-symptomatic (prodrome) phase to actual illness; and (3) investigate the genetic and biological mechanisms underlying SMI in order to understand how, in the future, we can preempt illness from ever occurring. Here are examples of NIMH efforts on these three fronts:

1. In the United States, the delay between a first episode of psychosis and onset of treatment ranges from 61 to 166 weeks, with an average of 110 weeks.[16] NIMH seeks to reduce that delay as much as possible, through continued support of the Recovery After an Initial Schizophrenia Episode (RAISE) project; a large-scale research project to explore whether using early and aggressive treatment will reduce the symptoms and prevent the gradual deterioration of functioning

that is characteristic of chronic schizophrenia. The project is currently focused on maintaining the quality of the treatment over time, and retaining individuals in treatment. Results from initial analyses suggest that a RAISE-type intervention would not only produce superior clinical outcomes, but will reduce re-hospitalization during the first year.
2. NIMH is continuing to fund research directed at the prodromal phase of schizophrenia, the stage just prior to full psychosis. A consortium of eight clinical research centers (North American Prodrome Longitudinal Study or NAPLS) are using biological assessments, including neuroimaging, electrophysiology, neurocognitive testing, hormonal assays, and genomics, to improve our ability to predict who will convert to psychosis, and to develop new approaches to pre-emptive intervention.
3. For decades, we have known that schizophrenia has a genetic component, but different methods for studying genetic changes have led to uncertainty about which genes are involved and how they contribute to illness. Using a new method to integrate information about illness-related genes from different types of studies, NIMH-supported researchers have identified a network of genes that affect the development, structure, and function of brain cells. The researchers detected important variations in how these gene-related brain changes affected risk for schizophrenia versus other disorders.[17]

## PREEMPTION: THE FUTURE OF MENTAL HEALTH RESEARCH

Research has taught us to detect diseases early and intervene quickly to preempt later stages of illness. This year we will avert 1.1 million deaths from heart disease because we have not waited for a heart attack to diagnose and treat coronary artery disease.[18] The 100,000 young Americans who will have a first episode of psychosis this year will join over two million with schizophrenia. Our best hope of reducing mortality from this, other SMI, and other brain disorders will come from realizing that just like other medical disorders, we need to diagnose and intervene before the symptoms become manifest. The health of the country cannot wait.

# End Notes

[1] Substance Abuse and Mental Health Services Administration. Results from the 2009 National Survey on Drug Use and Health: Mental Health Findings (Office of Applied Studies, NSDUH Series H-39, HHS Publication No. SMA 10-4609). Rockville, MD: Substance Abuse and Mental Health Services Administration, 2010.

[2] The World Health Organization. The global burden of disease: 2004 update, Table A2: Burden of disease in DALYs by cause, sex and income group in WHO regions, estimates for 2004. Geneva, Switzerland: WHO, 2008.

[3] Centers for Disease Control and Prevention, National Center for Injury Prevention and Control. Web-based Injury Statistics Query and Reporting System (WISQARS): www.cdc.gov/ncipc/wisqars accessed November 2011.

[4] Insel TR. Assessing the economic cost of serious mental illness. Am J Psychiatry. 2008 Jun;165(6):663-5.

[5] Soni A. The Five Most Costly Conditions, 1996 and 2006: Estimates for the U.S. Civilian Noninstitutionalized Population. Statistical Brief #248. July 2009. Agency for Healthcare Research and Quality, Rockville, MD.

[6] Bloom DE, Cafiero ET, Jané-Llopis E, Abrahams-Gessel S, Bloom LR, Fathima S, Feigl AB, Gaziano T, Mowafi M, Pandya A, Prettner K, Rosenberg L, Seligman B, Stein A, Weinstein C. The Global Economic Burden of Non-communicable Diseases. Geneva, Switzerland: World Economic Forum, 2011.

[7] Druss BG, Zhao L, Von Esenwein S, Morrato EH, Marcus SC. Understanding excess mortality in persons with mental illness: 17-year follow up of a nationally representative US survey. Med Care. 2011 Jun;49(6):599-604.

[8] Goff DC, Sullivan LM, McEvoy JP, et al. A comparison of ten-year cardiac risk estimates in schizophrenia patients from the CATIE study and matched controls. Schizophrenia Res. 2005;80(1):45-53.

[9] Allison DB, Fontaine KR, Heo M, et al. The distribution of body mass index among individuals with and without schizophrenia. J Clin Psych. 1999;60(4):215-220.

[10] McElroy SL. Correlates of overweight and obesity in 644 patients with bipolar disorder. J Clin Psych. 2002;63:207-213.

[11] McEvoy JP, Meyer JM, Goff DC, et al. Prevalence of the metabolic syndrome in patients with schizophrenia: Baseline results from the (CATIE) schizophrenia trial and comparison with national estimates from NHANES III. Schizophrenia Res. 2005;80(1):19-32.

[12] Hor K. & Taylor M. Suicide and schizophrenia: a systematic review of rates and risk factors. J Psychopharmacol. 2010;24(4S): 81-90.

[13] Wang PS, Berglund PA, Olfson M, Kessler RC. Delays in initial treatment contact after first onset of a mental disorder. Health Serv Res. 2004 Apr;39(2):393-415.

[14] Steadman HJ, Mulvey EP, Monahan J, Robbins PC, Appelbaum PS, Grisso T, Roth LH, Silver E. Violence by people discharged from acute psychiatric inpatient facilities and by others in the same neighborhoods. Arch Gen Psychiatry. 1998 May;55(5):393-401.

[15] Teplin, LA, McClelland, GM, Abram, KM & Weiner, DA. Crime victimization in adults with severe mental illness: comparison with the National Crime Victimization Survey. Arch Gen Psychiatry, 2005, 62(8), 911-921.

[16] Marshall M, Lewis S, Lockwood A, Drake R, Jones P, Croudace T. Association between duration of untreated psychosis and outcome in cohorts of first-episode patients. Arch Gen Psychiatry. 2005 Sep 62:975-983.

[17] Gilman SR, Chang J, Xu B, Bawa TS, Gogos JA, Karayiorgou M, Vitkup D. Diverse types of genetic variation converge on functional gene networks involved in schizophrenia. Nat Neurosci. 2012 Nov;15(12):1723-8.

[18] Vital Statistics of the United States, CDC/National Center for Health Statistics. (2011, August). Age-adjusted Death Rates for Coronary Heart Disease (CHD). National Heart Lung and Blood Institute. Retrieved January 23, 20130, from http://www.nhlbi.nih.gov/news/spotlight/success/conquering-cardiovascular-disease.html

*Chapter 4*

# TESTIMONY OF MICHAEL F. HOGAN, FORMER COMMISSIONER, NEW YORK STATE OFFICE OF MENTAL HEALTH. HEARING ON "ASSESSING THE STATE OF AMERICA'S MENTAL HEALTH SYSTEM"[*]

The mental health community appreciates the attention of the Committee, and the concern for consumers, families and providers that it represents. Mental health needs are substantial, but such attention from policy-makers is rare.

What is the state of the mental health system? A decade ago, a commission appointed by President George W. Bush to review mental health care told the president that despite the efforts of many dedicated people "the Unites States mental health services delivery system is in shambles." While many of the challenges we addressed still exist, problems and solutions are clearer a decade later. I hope we can provide you with a helpful picture of them.

*Much has changed, while much appears to remain the same.* The Nation's mental health system had its origins in the asylums of the 19th century. While much has been said about the balance between institutional and community care, a bigger issue is that for most of our history, mental health care has been separate from health care—and also unequal. In the best recent study of mental

---

[*] This is an edited, reformatted and augmented version of a testimony, presented January 24, 2013 before the Senate Committee on Health, Education, Labor, and Pensions.

health policy, Richard Frank and Sherry Glied assessed whether people with a mental illness were better off early in this century than 50 years earlier. They answered that question in the name of their monograph: *"Better, but not well."* However, the main insight from their study is that the improved well-being of people with a mental illness is not mainly due to changes within mental health care. Rather, the well-being of people with mental illness improved as they gained access to mainstream benefits like health care, disability insurance and housing. Improvements within the mental health system, like new treatments, had a smaller effect.

This trend has now accelerated. A major example is legislation known by the two outstanding Senators, a political odd couple united by concern for mental health, who sponsored it: Pete Dominici and Paul Wellstone. The 2007 passage of the *Mental Health Equity and Addictions Parity Act* (MHEAPA) was not about improvements within the mental health system. It was about including mental illness care in health care. It signaled that a separate and unequal mental health system was not an adequate solution.

Mental health care was also greatly enhanced by passage of the Patient *Protection and Affordable Care Act* (ACA). Building on Dominici-Wellstone, the ACA included mental health within its changes to health care. These two pieces of legislation are game changers for mental health. The inclusion of mental health will lead to profound changes that will play out over the next generation. Because health care is so complex and change is unpredictable, there will be false starts and dead ends. But any assessment of the state of America's mental health system must begin with a realization that we have begun to take big steps away from an approach that was both separate and unequal. The major challenges facing us are first whether including mental health in health care can be done sensibly, and second whether the portions of the mental health safety net that have value can be sustained. Inclusion creates big opportunities that we can seize or let slip away. In an earlier era of deinstitutionalization, we did not sustain our commitments to those most in need during change. Can we get it right this time?

*Integrating mental health care into health care.* A first major challenge for the next decade is to integrate basic mental health care into primary care. (Integrating primary medical care into mental health centers is also important, but not my major focus here.) We know that most Americans with mental health problems get no treatment for these problems. We also know that more people are treated by their family physician or other primary care practitioner than by mental health specialists. The problem is that we have many unmet needs while many specialty mental health programs are at capacity. The opportunity before us is that health coverage that includes mental health care will become available for many Americans. We must use this opportunity to provide integrated primary care that includes basic mental health care. There is less stigma in visits to primary care. People with a chronic illness like diabetes, cancer or hypertension who also have depression have health care costs at least 50% higher; and good basic mental health care reduces overall costs. Improving basic mental health care in primary care is a huge need and opportunity.

It will not occur automatically. Mental health care within primary care today is often inadequate. It can be done well, improving health and reducing costs, but barriers must be addressed. For example, "carved out" benefits for mental health care can usually be used only if a specialist is seen. Across primary care settings that have not upgraded to provide integrated care, less than half of the patients with a mental health problem get a mental illness diagnosis and treatment. Payments and supports for basic mental health care in primary care are often lacking, so less than 15% of the people with depression in primary care get adequate care. As a result, people with medical conditions like diabetes or high blood pressure as well as a mental health concern have bad health outcomes and higher medical costs.

We have an opportunity to address this problem because many people with these conditions will now have insurance that includes mental health care, and because practical ways to deliver basic mental health care in primary care settings are now well established. The approach, known as collaborative care, improves both health and mental health outcomes and also reduces total costs. Collaborative care is research tested and replicated in many real world clinics. The move to integrated care takes work, but its core elements are not complex: station a mental health practitioner in the practice, screen for mental health problems, measure progress, allow billing for basic mental health services like educating patients about managing their depression and ensure a psychiatrist or other specialist is available for consultation.

While collaborative care is proven, barriers to integrated care like separate benefits that are not available to primary care must be addressed. For collaborative care to work, the primary care setting must have its costs covered, including the modest additional costs of providing integrated care. There are also barriers in federal standards. Medicare still does not pay adequately for the elements of collaborative care, despite the terrible burden of depression and other mental health challenges for older Americans. National screening recommendations are also outdated. They say, in effect, "If you have plenty of resources to treat depression, you ought to screen for it." This is ridiculous. In my view, removing obstacles to primary care treatment of basic mental health problems is a core element of getting mental health parity right. It would be timely and very helpful if the Committee were to track progress toward integrated care.

*Protecting the safety net.* While health reform creates opportunities to improve care for many Americans, the safety net for individuals with the most serious mental illness is very stressed. This system, which evolved from state asylums and mental health centers to a diverse array of community based treatment, rehabilitation and support services, is directed and managed at the state and sometimes the county level. Its financing depends on Medicaid and state general funds. And given state budget shortfalls, resources have been cut. The National Association of State Mental Health Program Directors (NASMHPD) indicates that state mental health funding was reduced by more than $4B between 2009 and 2012.

While these cuts have been damaging, in many states the mental health safety net is stronger than it was a quarter century ago. Dedicated providers as well as state and local officials have learned what works. For example, we understand that decent, safe and affordable housing is a foundation for recovery, and a "Housing First" approach that first finds homeless mentally ill people a place to live and then assists with health and mental health has become a usual approach. We understand that people in recovery from mental illness and addiction working as "peer specialists" play an invaluable role as staff of community agencies. Many community mental health agencies are also integrating medical services into their mental health clinics, to address the co-occurring medical problems of the people they serve. So while the mental health safety net is stretched to the limits, it is better focused and more relevant than in the past.

There are threats to the safety net as health reform proceeds. Budget cuts have taken their toll, and we hope that as states move past budgets depleted by the recession there will not be further deep cuts. But there is also a concern about the erosion of informed leadership for the safety net system. Within states, as Medicaid has become the dominant payer for mental health services, the mantle of leadership is swinging away from mental health (and addiction) agencies toward Medicaid and Health agencies. A similar trend is occurring at the level where health care is managed; there is a movement toward managed care and within managed care there is movement from specialty behavioral health plans to mainstream managed care. The question is whether we can sustain the focus on quality of care for those most in need during this transition. We do not yet have national standards for the quality of care for people with serious mental illness, so the transition away from expert leadership is risky. We failed to maintain focus during an earlier era of deinstitutionalization; we must not make this mistake again.

*Children's mental health care.* Mental health problems have been called "the major chronic diseases of childhood." Mental illness usually emerges before young people enter high school, but the average lag to treatment is 9 years. Only about a quarter of children with mental health problems see a mental health professional, and often not enough care is delivered to make a difference. At the same time, we are scandalized by reports showing increased levels of psychiatric medication use among children, often with no adequate counseling to supplement or as alternative to medications. We see the results of insufficient mental health care in school failure and youth suicide. How do we do better?

While the gaps in children's mental health care are huge there is also reason for hope. In part, this is because we know more about what works, and what doesn't. We must start applying this knowledge. The timing is right if we act as we should; there are opportunities in healthcare reform and in calls to improve school mental health care. But like improvements to mental health care in primary care, improvement will not occur unless steps like these are taken:

- Make screening for and treating maternal depression standard for the first two years after birth. Maternal depression is prevalent, treatable, and can lead to big problems in development of the young child if left untreated. Treating mom's depression reduces levels of mental health problems for her children by half!
- Help pediatric practices and child mental health programs to provide holistic care. Noted columnist David Brooks—scarcely a bleeding heart liberal—has written persuasively of the problem of children growing up without the ability to "self regulate"—to manage themselves and their own behavior. These skills can be taught –but only if we begin early by providing structured support to young parents. To do this, we need to be able to:
    o Begin therapy for children without a specific diagnosis—to reduce the chance that a serious diagnosis will be given later.
    o Allow comprehensive pediatric practices and child mental health programs to bill for parent training and support for behavior management—to reduce the use of major medication use after the behavior has gotten worse

- o Reimburse and support team based care in pediatrics including physician attendance at team meetings with families
- o Reimburse pediatric and child mental health programs for carecoordination with schools and other agencies; care coordination may be
- o more effective and cost-effective than layering on additional treatments.
- Put better performance standards in place for child mental health programs. Right now national standards are limited to ADHD and follow up after hospitalization. Adolescent depression indicators are being developed but are not yet approved or used. What doesn't get measured in health care often doesn't get done.
- Do school mental health right. The President's proposals following the tragedy in Newtown include significant expansion of school mental health. Done right, this could be a significant benefit. But we now know more about what is effective, and what isn't. Expanded programs should only use proven approaches, such as peer-assisted learning, and cognitive behavioral interventions for trauma, adapted for schools. Each of these approaches has been linked to improving educational outcomes.

Develop a national approach for effective early treatment of psychotic illness. Our nation's approach to helping people with psychotic illnesses like schizophrenia is shameful. Usually, young people slip into psychotic illnesses for several years while they—or their families—get no help. When they have a "first psychotic break," they usually are briefly hospitalized. Almost always, medications take the worst of the symptoms away—within days or weeks. So then they are discharged with a referral to care and maybe a recommendation of a support group. This is woefully, stupidly deficient. Having symptoms reduced is not a cure. When people feel better, and especially since the drugs have significant side effects, they often stop taking them. Relapse is likely. Usually the second break is worse. And then the revolving door begins. Often after decades people figure out how to manage their illness, but by then they are often on permanent disability status, unemployed, and in terrible health.

Some have suggested that the solution to this problem is in going backward—not forward—to days when stays in mental hospitals were measured in months and years. This is idiotic. There is no research to suggest it is effective. It is terribly expensive. Hospitals cannot be run (as the old asylums were) on unpaid patient labor. And a civilized society cannot detain people on a vague hope they will get better. So we will not turn the clock back on mental health care. But we do need a modern approach to care for people with psychotic disorders, one that replaces both the asylum and the revolving door with continuous team treatment like that we provide for people with chronic medical problems. Teams delivering First Episode Psychosis (FEP) care have figured out how to do this work. It is person-centered, family driven, collaborative and recovery oriented. Staying in school or work is encouraged—though adaptations may be needed. It is time to implement this approach, as both Australia and Great Britain have done. We need not lag behind other nations in this area. Our country needs to make modest investments now to develop FEP teams so that families anywhere in the state struggling with a young adult who is slipping away from sanity can get good care reasonably close to home. The Committee's attention to this issue could have an enormous positive effect.

*Lifelong disability for people with mental illness is usually unnecessary.* While many of the worst outcomes of serious mental illness (e.g. homelessness, comorbid medical illness, incarceration) are receiving increased attention, we are failing systematically to help people escape poverty and disability. In effective supported employment approaches such as Individual Placement with Supports (IPS) a majority of adults with serious mental illness find a job. But we generally fail to use this effective program. The nation's Vocational Rehabilitation (VR) system is focused on employment for people with disabilities, but it is limited in scope and flawed in its approach to helping people with mental illness. Most people with serious mental illness never get VR services, and among those who do, outcomes are worse than for other groups of people with disabilities. Most VR programs do not use IPS systematically. Meanwhile, Medicaid does not pay for key components of IPS. Because of these cracks between systems, an effective approach is usually not made available, and the employment rate among people with serious mental illness who are receiving care is, scandalously, about 15%.

Supplemental Security Income (SSI) and, for those who become disabled after working, Social Security Disability Income (SSDI) are invaluable lifelines for people with serious disability including serious mental illness. But many people with mental illness on SSDI and SSI want to work. And most could work—at the very least in part-time private sector employment— if IPS was available and if disability was not an "all or nothing" program.

I would like to bring to the Committee's attention an innovative program established by New York State and the Social Security Administration to address this problem. It takes advantage of Ticket To Work—a well-intended back-to-work incentive program that has never reached its potential, largely because of its complexity. The New York State Office of Mental Health (OMH) in collaboration with the New York Department of Labor and other state agencies serving people with disabilities developed a comprehensive employment system for people with serious mental illness and other disabilities. Key components include: 1) education and counseling on benefits (such as how to maintain Medicaid coverage while working, and how to take advantage of complex Social Security work incentives); 2) an integrated information system that links people to and is built onto the Department of Labor's workforce system; and 3) a statewide network of IPS services delivered through OMH Personalized Recovery Oriented Services (PROS) programs. Via a unique partnership agreement, the Social Security Administration has designated this system including all participating consumers and providers as a Ticket To Work *Employment Network*. This arrangement is the most systematic statewide approach to employment services and to fully using available benefits to support productivity instead of poverty and disability.

I urge the Committee's attention to the costs and consequences of unnecessary disability for people with serious mental illness, in particular to:

- Assuring that Vocational Rehabilitation and Medicaid figure out how to make effective Individual Placement with Supports services available to all people with serious mental illness who want work instead of poverty, and
- How the Social Security/New York partnership can be implemented in other states.

*Suicide prevention*: Now is the time to act. We are dismayed by reports that deaths by suicide in the Armed Forces last year exceeded other combat deaths. This concern is surely justified. Yet this is but the tip of the iceberg; twice as many American lives are lost to suicide in the average week than to military suicide in a year. Suicide, which is the tenth leading cause of death – and the third leading cause of death among young adults—receives a relatively small investment in terms of research and programming than other public health problems of its magnitude. We can and we must do more.

The administration, to its credit, has begun to focus on suicide prevention. In 2010, Secretaries Sebelius and Gates launched the Action Alliance on Suicide Prevention, a public-private partnership co-chaired by Army Secretary John McHugh and former Senator Gordon Smith. With support from the

Action Alliance, Surgeon General Regina Benjamin has released a comprehensive update of the National Strategy on Suicide Prevention, originally released in 2001. Yet more action is needed. Suicide prevention activities are scattered and thin. Outside the Department of Defense, the only national efforts are the National Suicide Prevention Lifeline (1- 800-273-TALK), a technical assistance center, and the small network of youth and college prevention programs funded by the Substance Abuse and Mental Health Services Administration under the Garrett Lee Smith Memorial Youth Suicide Prevention Act.

It is time to do more to fight this needless and often preventable form of death. It is claiming the lives of students, soldiers, veterans, and Americans of every age and background. Congressional action would help advance this cause, as it did with passage of the Garrett Lee Smith Act. The Action Alliance is focusing integrating state-of the-science suicide prevention practices into initiatives under the Affordable Care Act. We assess that current clinical practices in the U.S. are one to two decades behind the research, which demonstrates that effective care, what we call "suicide care," targeted to patients who are at risk, can significantly improve their prognosis. The Affordable Care Act offers numerous opportunities to incorporate best and effective practices into preventive services offered through Medicare and Medicaid, into electronic health records, and into other reform initiatives.

Suicide prevention is an area where small amounts of money can make a difference. The Action Alliance has the potential to bend the curve on suicide, but it is funded this year via a time-limited grant from SAMHSA. Similarly, the Nation's network of certified crisis lines, although linked together by the SAMHSA funded Lifeline project, is mostly funded by state and local-level grants and philanthropy, yet it is projected to respond to a million callers this year, a large proportion of whom are in utter desperation and on the threshold of their own death. Research has conclusively shown that these crisis lines are effective and are performing as an indispensable part of the nation's health care system, yet they receive no federal support. The Committee's attention could help assure that other federal agencies do more to help, that the National Action Alliance for Suicide Prevention is sustained and that the national network of crisis lines is strengthened. These steps would be life-saving.

*Conclusion.* We thank the Committee again for focusing on mental health needs and opportunities, and we hope our suggestions are relevant and helpful. Some of the issues I discuss do not necessarily suggest easy fixes. But mental health concerns are coming out of the shadows, at a time of major change in health and mental health care. Now is the time to get it right. We face major opportunities to improve health care for millions of Americans, but these are opportunities that can easily be missed. Similarly, we cannot allow what remains of the nation's mental health system for people with the most serious disorders to be dissipated. In an earlier, failed era of deinstitutionalization, patients were dumped into unprepared communities. This is not the time to dump them again, into "mainstream" arrangements without adequate protections and accountabilities. Fixing the mental health system requires more than gun control. And it is possible.

In: U.S. Mental Health Workforce ...
Editor: Maurice Gordon

ISBN: 978-1-62948-865-3
© 2014 Nova Science Publishers, Inc.

*Chapter 5*

# TESTIMONY OF DR. BOB VERO, CEO, CENTERSTONE OF TENNESSEE. HEARING ON "ASSESSING THE STATE OF AMERICA'S MENTAL HEALTH SYSTEM"[*]

On behalf of Centerstone, I would like to personally thank Senator Alexander and Senator Harkin for the opportunity to comment on the state of the U.S. Mental Health System from the community mental health perspective. I hope what I share will assist the Health, Education, Labor and Pensions Committee as you seek to gain an understanding of opportunities to address the gaps and barriers within our mental healthcare system.

To work in the area of community mental health is, without question, an extraordinary privilege. It is likewise a tremendous responsibility.

I have been fortunate throughout my career to participate in and observe our field from different perspectives—as a clinician, a critical incident responder, faculty member, research collaborator, client, and as a CEO. I have worked with hoarders whose homes were so cluttered that there was no longer safe passage to their beds for rest and refrigerators so contaminated that the contents were no longer safe to consume. I have worked with people who are so profoundly disturbed they've committed despicable and sometimes illegal acts. My role with these patients was to quell their psychosis and ensure safety for themselves and others. I also have had the responsibility of treating a

---

[*] This is an edited, reformatted and augmented version of a testimony presented January 24, 2013 before the Senate Committee on Health, Education, Labor, and Pensions.

mother's depression and complex grief following the tragic death of her preschool-aged child.

I have seen first-hand what the research shows – mental illness truly affects everyone. One in four American adults will have a diagnosable mental illness in any given year, and about one in 17 adults, 6% of the population, have a serious mental illness.[1]

As a community mental health center (CMHC), we are entrusted with the care of individuals, families, and communities whose lives have been impacted by mental illness. As health care leaders, we are called upon to work to create a mental healthcare system rooted in compassion, scientific understanding, individual recovery and, ultimately, disease management, prevention and cure.

I chose this field nearly four decades ago because I thought that effective treatment for mental illness could have an equal or even more profound impact on families than treatment for heart disease and cancer. In school, I saw my inspired, intelligent friends devastated by anxiety, depression and bipolar disorder. I witnessed how trauma could weaken even the strongest of my colleagues.

Over the years, I have found this to be true in my own family as well, especially when my forty-year old cousin, Lisa, took her own life. I wish she had been able to ask for help when her pain became unbearable because I know there is an alternative to senseless death. Mental health treatment is life-saving.

## ROLE OF COMMUNITY MENTAL HEALTH CENTERS

Community mental health centers have an incredibly important role to help provide effective, high quality care to the children, families, and older adults they serve. We help to keep children together with their families. We provide a lifeline for people struggling at all levels of severity of need, from mild levels of anxiety to acute episodes of depression to those contemplating suicide. Our treatment services and broad array of services for all ages, work to prevent horrible tragedies while helping to build strong, healthy, resilient communities. Community mental health centers, as a whole, fill a tremendous gap and, moreover, do a tremendous job for the people we serve. There are, nevertheless, several significant barriers and gaps in the current U.S. mental health system that make it difficult for our local agencies to serve as the community safety net they were envisioned to be 50 years ago by President Kennedy.

## BARRIERS AND GAPS IN ACCESS TO HIGH QUALITY CHILD AND ADOLESCENT SERVICES

One of the biggest barriers is a lack of access to services for children and youth. Sadly, due to a lack of a federal definition of what services a community mental center should offer, many towns and cities, especially rural ones, do not have access to a safety net provider, offering a full continuum of evidence-based services to children and youth within a service area. Since 50% of mental illnesses start before the age of 14, and three out of four people develop their condition, including bipolar disorder, depression and schizophrenia by young adulthood, this lack of access can have tragic, lasting effects.[2] We know from the research that the right care at the right time has a huge potential to reduce the occurrence of mental illnesses, the severity of those illnesses, and their impact on people's lives. Early mental health interventions for young children and families can reduce risk factors for mental illness and increase protective factors that build resiliency.[3] If children impacted by multiple traumatic experiences do not get the care they need, it can have serious, life-long consequences.[4]

There are several ways to address this barrier:

- The most permanent fix would be to pass language similar to that included within the Excellence in Mental Health Act specifically defining that a community mental health center has to provide a full continuum of services across the lifespan – including early intervention services.
- Grant funding streams that encourage existing centers to expand their service continuum and partner with community organizations are also helpful. At Centerstone, due to grant funding from SAMHSA and the Department of Education, we have been able to offer mental health and substance abuse services within rural schools for children and youth. We are now co-located in 160 preschools, middle and high schools throughout Tennessee, serving as adjunct faculty and providing a service to the school, they would likely be unable to deliver without our partnership. In addition, we recently were awarded a grant for early intervention services for families of infants and toddlers at risk for emotional problems
- Pass Health IT legislation so that community mental health centers, especially rural centers, can access telehealth services. With a severe

and growing national shortage of child, adolescent, and adult psychiatrists,5 telehealth is one of the key ways to foster improved access to services for children and adults with serious mental illness, especially in underserved and rural areas.

## BARRIERS TO ENGAGING THE WHOLE FAMILY IN CARE

For our children, the most effective care involves treating the entire family. Over and over, my staff, who work with children in schools and other community settings, share frustrations and concerns for the children they treat because of limited or entirely no access to the child's parents or caregivers. So often we detect issues in parents and other people in the child's environment, yet we are sometimes hindered in our ability to treat the entire family unit due to inadequate insurance coverage. There are barriers to treating their uninsured or underinsured parents who have their own mental health needs and issues. We need to be able to teach parenting skills if we want the child's behavior to change. We need to be able to address the parent's depression or addiction if we want to make an impact on a child's anxiety, truancy, or aggression. A mother is only able to advocate for her child and coordinate care if she, herself is healthy and able to cope. We are eagerly awaiting further news regarding a decision related to Medicaid expansion. It will allow community mental health centers to treat the low income parent's depression, substance use disorder, and/or other condition that impede effective parenting.

Research shows that programs that engage the whole family, whether teaching parenting skills in a clinic or modeling those skills in a home setting is effective in reducing aggression, disruptive and antisocial behavior, and preventing substance abuse later in life.[6] With SAMHSA grant funding, Centerstone has been able to implement these interventions in different communities in Tennessee, resulting in some incredible outcomes. However, sustainability often remains a barrier once grant-funding concludes.

## GAPS BETWEEN DIFFERENT CARE PROVIDING SYSTEMS

We hear a lot about America's fragmented health care system with current news focusing on mental health care. Children with serious emotional disturbances and mental disorders and their parents, in order to get the care they need, often have multiple providers and interface with multiple agencies (i.e. department of children's services, juvenile justice, pediatric office, school, mental health center, etc.) The consequence is at best costly, and at worst dangerous. Care coordination models have proven effective outcomes. We encourage the expansion of these evidence-based models. There is an opportunity here for greater collaboration and shared accountability by mandating mental health and substance abuse services be incorporated into the clinical models funded by the Affordable Care Act.

## TRANSITIONS IN YOUNG ADULT CARE

Currently, when many adolescents with mental illness reach adulthood, they are at risk for experiencing a disruption in care if their state's Medicaid plan does not have an eligibility class or allowance for an "aging out" transition plan. Even though the ACA affords insurance coverage for dependents, up to the age of 26 years old, on their parent insurance plans, many youth will not have access to such coverage. This issue must be addressed as states consider plans for Medicaid expansion.

## EXCLUSION OF COMMUNITY MENTAL HEALTH CENTERS FROM HITECH ACT

Thanks to the work of the Office of the National Coordinator for Health IT and the leadership of Sen. Sheldon Whitehouse, there have been tremendous advances towards creating standardized guidelines. However, since community mental health centers were left out of the 2009 HITECH Act, we have not been able to fully benefit from these advances. This one barrier sets up roadblocks for the achievement of several key goals for our field. If behavioral health were included in this Act, we would be positioned to:

- Effectively share information for purposes of coordination of care, including treatment plans, with primary providers, integrating our work to the benefit of the patient.
- Preventing overprescribing and other consequences of failed drug coordination such as drug-drug interaction and/or toxicity.
- Effectively track outcomes over time.

From the CMHC perspective, I do not know how centers can ensure that the care we are providing is what we would want for each of our family members without using Health IT tools. The first 25 years I spent in this field were with paper records, and I can tell you the difference between clinical supervision of paper records and clinical supervision using analytics tools is night and day. Thanks to the Ayers Foundation and the Joe C Davis Foundation, Centerstone was able to develop analytics tools similar to those used by for-profit businesses. With these tools, I can hotspot clinics, locations and centers where outcomes are lagging and rapidly develop localized quality improvement plans. I can ask questions, like "how many children are we serving in foster care and have been prescribed atypical antipsychotic medications in the last three months," or "how is our HEDIS client engagement metric last month compared to last year" and get the answer in one short minute.

As primarily Medicaid providers, most community mental health centers exist with very little financial margin, if any. Funding large health IT purchases is a luxury most cannot afford. Due to the contrary, due to the billions in cuts our field has experienced over the last four years, some community mental health centers have been forced to simply shut their doors while many more have quietly ended programs and laid off large numbers of employees.

Inadequate Health IT capacity impedes the ability of the whole field to improve the quality of mental health care. Centers not using Health IT are, moreover, unable to use analytics tools to look at quality metrics or conduct rapid, targeted quality audits.

Most health information exchanges do not include community mental health centers, and many states have no regulations allowing the sharing of information electronically with CMHCs. Systems and processes designed to foster provider communications and shared data through electronic means would greatly improve health care outcomes and reduce cost.

Strong bipartisan bills in both houses of Congress would correct this problem. HR 6043 championed by Representatives Tim Murphy of Pennsylvania and Marsha Blackburn of Tennessee and S. 539 introduced by Senators Whitehouse and Collins would authorize the participation of mental health and addiction providers in the healthcare revolution sparked by passage of the HITECH Act in 2009.

## NEED FOR FORMAL MENTAL HEALTH CRISIS SERVICES IN EVERY COMMUNITY

Not all states, counties, and community mental health centers offer formal crisis response services. Whether by telephone, internet, text or in-person, having a system of trained professionals for immediate response in the event of a crisis is, simply put, life-saving. I am in support of the President's recommendation to increase mental health first aid training. I believe that it makes sense for every teacher, law enforcement officer, and first responder in the U.S. to know how to detect issues and engage someone to get help. However, we need to make sure that as we are training people to seek help when in crisis, we have an existing network available to respond to the situation and provide evidence-based, outcomes-driven services. It is not enough to detect an issue; someone must be able to respond.

The Excellence in Mental Health Act, as part of its definition for what a community mental health center should do, requires that it provide crisis services. From my perspective, I know that this service not only saves life, it saves dollars, and I encourage this be considered vital to the service continuum of mental health safety net centers. In 2012, our Tennessee Crisis Call Center handled 18,350 emergency calls. Our Mobile Crisis therapists provided 6,081 face-to-face crisis assessments and in doing so prevented over 3,000 mental health-related hospitalizations – a huge cost savings for our state Medicaid program. Our Mobile Crisis team also aided in the appropriate hospitalization of another 3,000 individuals whose acute needs required a level of care beyond traditional outpatient services. Although this might not have saved Medicaid funds, it likely prevented countless tragedies.

Tennessee's TennCare Director and Deputy Commissioner for the state department of Finance and Administration, Darin Gordon as with our Commissioner of Mental Health and Substance Abuse Services, Douglas Varney should be recognized for their support of a formal, statewide Crisis Services program, serving the acute psychiatric needs of all Tennesseans.

## NEED FOR INTEGRATED CARE

The quality and length of life of our patients requires that we accurately assess and effectively treat their physical as well as their mental health needs. Mental health and physical health are as intricately intertwined as the brain is to the body. There is ample evidence that the current fragmented system with one part of the health care field treating mental illness and one treating physical illness is costly and, moreover, ineffective.

While community mental health services are an extremely small percentage when you look at state budgets, mental disorders are one of the five most costly conditions in the United States.[7] Fifty-two percent of Dual Eligible beneficiaries with disabilities have a psychiatric illness. Psychiatric illness is found in three of the top five most expensive diagnosis dyads.[8] In a study of the fee for service Medi-Cal system in California, when the 11 percent of the Medi-Cal enrollees with a serious mental illness (SMI) in the study were compared with all Medi-Cal enrollees, the SMI group's spending was 3.7 times higher than the total population ($14,365 per person per year compared with $3,914).[9] They also had a higher prevalence of other costly health disorders (diabetes, heart disease, chronic respiratory disease).

Nationally, one in eight visits to emergency departments is due to mental disorders, a substance use disorder, or both.[10] All of this healthcare, while costly, has not resulted in better outcomes. People with serious mental illnesses, on average, die 25 years earlier than people without such diagnoses, and this early mortality is primarily due to preventable physical health conditions.[11]

Community mental health centers are key to improving physical health while simultaneously lowering health care costs. The same skills we use to prevent mental health hospitalizations can be used to prevent physical health hospitalizations. The same skills our clinicians use to promote behavior changes in depressive cognitive thought patterns or patients with alcoholism can be used to help our patients quit smoking, exercise more, and make healthy food choices. The same nurses in our clinics that test for lithium and clozapine blood levels could test for hemoglobin A1C levels and draw lipid screens. The same case managers that do home visits and check on whether someone with schizophrenia is taking their medication and meeting their mental health goals also could teach the patient how to take their blood pressure and track their weight. Our expertise in behavior change is part of the solution to meet the triple aim of healthcare – reduced cost, improved health, and quality care. However, reimbursement for these activities varies depending on the Medicaid, Medicare and the managed care plan. Most CMHCs lack funds for training costs to train our staff, update our clinics, and obtain health IT systems that are compatible with primary care systems.

Thankfully, in 2009, SAMHSA launched its Primary Care and Mental Health Care Integration (PBHCI) program. This program seeks to improve the physical health status of people with serious mental illnesses and reduce their total health care costs through integration of services. SAMHSA has funded 94 sites nationally, and, in cooperation with HRSA, has co-funded a national resource center helping community mental health centers like Centerstone and Federally Qualified Health Centers and other primary care practices to integrate physical and behavioral health care.

This funding stream has been very welcomed by Centerstone. Centerstone of Indiana was part of the second cohort to receive funds. My organization, Centerstone of Tennessee, was part of the 5th cohort. The biggest barrier to making integrated care sustainable for community mental health remains funding restrictions. Thankfully, we have seen more openness to lift those restrictions from managed care companies and states, and we are hopeful that this will be changing rapidly.

More direction from CMS (Centers for Medicaid and Medicare Services) to states regarding definition of what services can and should be provided by mental health organizations might be helpful to make sure those restrictions lift. The Primary Care Mental Health Care Integration program is most valuable if it is sustainable, and sustainability can be achieved by some common sense changes.

## NEED FOR ADEQUATE AND CONSISTENT COVERAGE IN ACA

Currently, there is no guidance issued ensuring that behavioral health has a seat at the table for Accountable Care Organizations (ACO) and other care coordination models being adopted across the U.S. It would be helpful, in the final Affordable Care Act (ACA) guidelines, for Congress to set forth instructions for the coverage of mental health and substance abuse services in the care and coverage models established by the ACA.

## CONCLUSION

Recently, our country suffered a devastating loss of 28 precious lives – the 20 innocents, the 6 courageous teachers and administrators, the life of a mentally ill young man who did not get the care he needed, and the life of his mother, who did not get the help and information she needed. This tragedy, along with those in Colorado, Arizona, California, Virginia, and others has thrown a spotlight on our mental health system.

We have a long way to go to reach the President's vision of "making access to mental health care as easy as access to a gun." Our case managers, therapists, psychiatrists, nurses, researchers, and peer counselors are passionate about providing the best mental health care possible, and we seek to be part of the solution. However, we cannot achieve this solution in isolation. This is a moment that demands courage and action. Everyone in this room shares a responsibility for the future of mental health. Community mental health centers stand ready to work with you to improve the U.S. mental health system.

Thank you for your time and attention.

## End Notes

[1] Kessler RC, Chiu WT, Demler O, Walters EE. Prevalence, severity, and comorbidity of twelve-month DSM-IV disorders in the National Comorbidity Survey Replication (NCS-R). Archives of General Psychiatry, 2005 Jun; 62(6):617-27.

[2] Kessler, R. C., Berglund, P., Demler, O., et al. (2005). Lifetime prevalence and age-of-onset distributions of DSM-IV disorders in the National Comorbidity Survey replication. Archives of General Psychiatry, 62, 593-602.

[3] National Research Council and Institute of Medicine. (2011) Preventing Mental, Emotional, and Behavioral Disorders Among Young People: Progress and Possibilities. Committee on the Prevention of Mental Disorders and Substance Abuse Among Children, Youth, and Young Adults: Research Advances and Promising Interventions. Mary Ellen O'Connell, Thomas Boat, and Kenneth E. Warner, Editors. Board on Children, Youth, and Families, Division of Behavioral and Social Sciences and Education. Washington, DC: National Academies Press.

[4] Edwards VJ, Holden GW, Anda RF, Felitti VJ. Experiencing multiple forms of childhood maltreatment and adult mental health: results from the Adverse Childhood Experiences (ACE) Study . American Journal of Psychiatry 2003;160(8):1453–1460.

[5] American Academy of Child and Adolescent Psychiatry (AACAP). (2008) Analysis of American Medical Association Physician Masterfile. Washington, D.C.: American Academy of Child and Adolescent Psychiatry.

[6] National Research Council and Institute of Medicine. (2011) IBID.

[7] Agency for Healthcare Research and Quality (2013). AHRQ Program Brief: Mental Health Research Findings. Retrieved on January 19, 2013 from http://www.ahrq.gov/ research/ mentalhth.htm.

[8] Kronick RG, Bella M, Gilmer TP. (2009) The faces of Medicaid III: Refining the portrait of people with multiple chronic conditions. Center for Health Care Strategies, Inc.

[9] California 1115 Waiver Behavioral Health Technical Work Group. (2010). Beneficiary risk management: Prioritizing high risk SMI patients for case management/coordination. Presentation by JEN Associates, Cambridge, MA.

[10] Coffey R, et. al. (2010). Emergency Department Use for Mental and Substance Use Disorders. AHRQ.

[11] Parks J, Svendsen D, Singer P, Foti ME. (2006). Morbidity and Mortality in People with Serious Mental Illness. Alexandria, VA: National Association of State Mental Health Program Directors.

*Chapter 6*

# TESTIMONY OF LARRY FRICKS, SENIOR CONSULTANT, NATIONAL COUNCIL FOR COMMUNITY BEHAVIORAL HEALTHCARE. HEARING ON "ASSESSING THE STATE OF AMERICA'S MENTAL HEALTH SYSTEM"[*]

Good morning. Thank you, Chairman Harkin and Senator Alexander, for inviting me to speak at today's hearing. My name is Larry Fricks. I am a senior consultant to the National Council for Community Behavioral Healthcare and Deputy Director of the SAMHSA-HRSA Center for Integrated Health Solutions. I'd like to cover three topics today: first, the ongoing stigma and discrimination that surrounds behavioral health disorders and the need for better public education regarding the facts about mental illness and addiction; second, the critical role of peer support to promote recovery; and third, the importance of a whole health approach when it comes to improving our healthcare system.

As former First Lady Rosalynn Carter said, "stigma is the most damaging factor in the life of anyone who has a mental illness." Stigma is our biggest challenge.

Allow me to share with you today some of my lived experience of recovery from mental illness and substance abuse over the last 28 years,

---

[*] This is an edited, reformatted and augmented version of a testimony, presented January 24, 2013 before the Senate Committee on Health, Education, Labor, and Pensions.

focusing on peer support and the skills I learned to self-manage my mind-body health. As anyone who has experienced a mental health or substance use condition can tell you, we must fight a battle on two fronts: one against the diagnosis itself, and the other against public ignorance. According to data from the Substance Abuse and Mental Health Services Administration (SAMHSA),[1] one in five Americans will experience a mental health issue during any given year. Yet, as a society, we largely remain ignorant about the signs and symptoms of mental illness, and we ignore our role as supportive community members to help people experiencing these illnesses.

My grandmother, Naomi Brewton, graduated from the top of her class in college. But when she gave birth to her youngest son, she suffered what was then called a "nervous breakdown." Her father was Dr. Brewton, founder of Brewton-Parker College near Vidalia, Georgia. The stigma and ignorance around mental illness prompted the family to secretly send her off to North Carolina for treatment. When she returned, she was a different person. For all the years that I knew her, she was a total recluse, never leaving home.

My grandmother told great stories and had an infectious laugh that I loved, but I was never fully able to understand her life of tormented isolation until I was hospitalized three times in the mid-eighties. During my last hospitalization, I was kept in seclusion and restrained in my bed. When I returned home I sank into deep despair, overwhelmed by pending divorce, near financial collapse, and a weight gain of some 60 pounds from psychiatric medications. I internalized the stigma and discrimination experienced from mental illness, growing a negative self-image and sense of hopelessness from the prognosis that my life was over as I knew it, and thinking that highly society-valued roles like work may now be too stressful to consider. Like my grandmother, I began to isolate, with suicide becoming an attractive option.

Mounting research shows that people without a social network of support and a sense of meaning and purpose are less resilient against illness - mind and body - and often die younger. That's why meaningful work and peer support are emerging as huge factors in recovery and longevity. But in addition to peer support and gaining meaning and purpose from employment, my self-management really strengthened when I moved into mind-body resiliency. My life was forever changed after hearing a presentation by Dr. Fred Goodwin, former director of the National Institute of Mental Health and a specialist in bipolar illness. His research showed that restful sleep was a huge factor in building resiliency and preventing manic episodes like I had experienced. An anchor for my recovery is managing my sleep and reducing stress by practicing the Relaxation Response made famous by Dr. Herbert Benson at the Benson-

Henry Institute for Mind Body Medicine at Massachusetts General Hospital. I was fortunate to have a psychiatrist who fully supported focusing my recovery around managing my sleep and after doing so, changed my medication to help shed much of the weight I had gained.

Today, I live the kind of full and meaningful life that my grandmother was denied, because I was able to receive mental health services with a focus on recovery and learn self-management skills. We have come so far in the fight against stigma, in part because of greater public awareness and education about the nature of mental illness. You heard from another presenter about a program called Mental Health First Aid that teaches a five-step action plan to recognize the signs and symptoms of mental illness, respond to a person in crisis, and encourage seeking professional help, self-help and other support strategies. I am a Mental Health First Aid trainer, which means I teach people how to instruct others in becoming certified Mental Health First Aiders. I have witnessed first-hand the positive impact that comes from people with lived experience of recovery gaining the skills for providing support to help others experience a life of recovery from mental illness and substance abuse. MHFA attendees also learn about the growing awareness of the impact of trauma, especially childhood trauma, on mind-body health and why we need trauma-informed services and supports.

Members of the Committee, I urge you to support Mental Health First Aid and other public education programs that help Americans learn how to reach out to their friends and family members who may be experiencing a behavioral health condition. One bill to this effect has already been introduced in the House: The Mental Health First Aid Act (H.R. 274). I encourage you to give this bill a hearing when it is introduced in the Senate and offer your support when it comes before your committee this year.

Next, I would like to share some information about the newest workforce in behavioral health, called certified peer specialists. Peer specialists are trained in skills to promote strength-based recovery and whole health, delivering services that are Medicaid billable when included in state plans. Research on the effectiveness of peers in promoting recovery has been so positive that in 2007 the Centers for Medicare and Medicaid Services (CMS) issued guidelines for states wanting to bill for peer support services, proclaiming them "an evidence-based mental health model of care which consists of a qualified peer support provider who assists individuals with their recovery from mental illness and substance abuse disorders."[2]

Peer support specialists have personally addressed stigma and discrimination and gained the lived experience to promote recovery and support rather than illness and disability. Because of this, peer specialists are unique in their ability to connect with other peers to ignite hope and teach skills for recovery self-management and promoting whole health. According to a 2008 study by Eiken and Campbell, "The growing evidence includes reduced hospitalizations, reduced use of crisis services, improved symptoms, larger social support networks, and improved quality of life, as well as strengthening the recovery of the people providing the services."[3] Published 2006 research by Davidson et al., found that "peer providers can increase empowerment, decrease substance abuse, reduce days in the hospital, and increase use of outpatient services, at least as long as long as the peer support continues."[4] A 2006 study by Sells, et al, found "the unique role of trusted peers connecting with each other to foster hope and build on strengths is emerging as a key transformational factor in mental health services."[5]

One of the most innovative services beginning to spring up across the country are peer respite centers. Georgia funds three of these centers and they are proving highly effective at reducing hospitalizations, an important outcome the state has pledged to achieve under a Department of Justice settlement resulting from deaths in state hospitals. In Georgia, if a peer senses early warning signs of possible relapse, he or she can spend up to seven nights at a respite center supported by peer specialists promoting mind-body health and self-management. Georgia also recently received CMS approval for peer specialists certified in a new training created by the SAMHSA-HRSA Center for Integrated Health Solutions called Whole Health Action Management (WHAM) to bill Medicaid for peer whole health and wellness services.

I urge the Committee to support including certified peer specialists as billable providers under Medicaid, given their effective role in supporting their peers in recovery and whole health. However, because Medicaid requires "medical necessity" documenting illness and symptoms and peer specialists are trained to focus on strengths and supports, we need more flexible funding sources to grow the recovery and whole health outcomes peer support services can deliver.

This brings me to the final point I'd like to discuss today: the importance of addressing the mind-body connection when it comes to healthcare.

There can be no health without mental health. Conversely, we cannot successfully care for people with mental health and addiction disorders without addressing their co-occurring physical health disorders. Research indicates that people with severe mental illness in the U.S. who are served in the public healthcare system have an average life expectancy that is 25 years less than the general public. That's the same as the overall U.S. life expectancy in 1915, a time before any of the healthcare advances that have allowed us to lead steadily longer lives over the last century.

The primary culprits behind this shocking situation are untreated but preventable diseases that commonly occur together with mental illness and addictions: cardiovascular disease, diabetes, complications from smoking and some of side effects of psychiatric medications that cause weight gain and diabetes. Most people receive routine preventive care that would help identify these conditions early, make lifestyle changes, or receive appropriate medications to ensure they are well controlled. But people with serious mental illness often cannot access this preventive care – or even get treatment for their other health conditions.

The Substance Abuse and Mental Health Services Administration is working to rectify this problem by providing grants to community behavioral health centers for offering basic primary care screenings and coordinating referrals to primary care. As part of the Primary Care-Behavioral Health Integration program (PBHCI), nurses, trained care managers, peer specialists, and other types of healthcare professionals are now actively working in 94 grantee sites to screen patients for weight gain, blood lipid levels, cholesterol, and more.

Although data is still being collected, early results indicate that this program has been successful in helping people with behavioral health conditions maintain or reduce their weight, cholesterol, blood sugar, and other risk factors for chronic disease. I strongly urge the committee to support this important grant program.

In closing, I would like to say that nearly three decades of experience in behavioral health has taught me that the greatest potential for promoting recovery and whole health comes from within an individual, with the support of peers, family and community. My recommendation is to establish and support programs that drive this potential, putting the person at the center of all services, building on their strengths and supports.

## End Notes

[1] Substance Abuse and Mental Health Services Administration, Results from the 2011 National Survey on Drug Use and Health: Mental Health Findings, NSDUH Series H-45, HHS Publication No. (SMA) 12-4725. Rockville, MD: Substance Abuse and Mental Health Services Administration, 2012.

[2] Center for Medicare and Medicaid Services, State Medicaid Director Letter #07-011. August 15, 2007.

[3] Eiken, S., & Campbell, J. (2008). Medicaid coverage of peer support for people with mental illness: Available research and state example. Published by Thomson Reuters Healthcare. Retrieved from: http://cms.hhs.gov/PromisingPractices/downloads/PeerSupport.pdf

[4] Davidson, L., Chinman, M., Sells, D., & Rowe, M. (2006). Peer supports among adults with serious mental illness: A report from the field. Schizophrenia Bulletin, 32, 443-450.

[5] Sells, D., Davidson, L., Jewell, C., Faizer, P., & Rowe, M. (2006). The treatment relationship in peer-based and regular case management services for clients with severe mental illnesses. Psychiatric Services, 57(8): 1179-1184.

*Chapter 7*

# TESTIMONY OF GEORGE DELGROSSO, EXECUTIVE DIRECTOR, COLORADO BEHAVIORAL HEALTH COUNCIL. HEARING ON "ASSESSING THE STATE OF AMERICA'S MENTAL HEALTH SYSTEM"[*]

Chairman Harkin and Sen. Alexander, thanks for giving me the opportunity to appear before the Senate HELP Committee on behalf of the Colorado Behavioral Healthcare Council and the National Council for Behavioral Health. My name is George DelGrosso and I am the Chief Executive Officer of the Colorado Behavioral Health Council (CBHC).

The CBHC is a statewide organization composed of 28 behavioral health organizations including all of the 17 Community Mental Health Centers, 2 specialty mental health clinics, 4 managed service organizations and 5 behavioral health organizations. The latter organizations are the management entities throughout the state for substance use disorder and the State's Medicaid mental health managed care program.

Our members provide psychiatric care, intensive community-based services and addiction treatment to over 120,000 Coloradans each year. About 50% of our mental health center consumer/patient caseload is composed of adults with severe mental illnesses like schizophrenia and bipolar disorder. We also serve children with serious mental and emotional disturbances referred to

---

[*] This is an edited, reformatted and augmented version of a testimony, presented January 24, 2013 before the Senate Committee on Health, Education, Labor, and Pensions.

us by their families, the Colorado juvenile justice, special education and foster care systems.

I will be devoting the bulk of my testimony today to the Colorado Mental Health First Aid program because we believe that it's an exciting new public health approach to early identification of mental illnesses and other mental health disorders. You will hear other witnesses testify today that mental disorders often begin manifesting themselves by as early as 14 years of age. According the American Psychiatric Association Diagnostic and Statistical Manual, the first obvious symptoms of severe mental illnesses occur between ages 18 and 24. But, on average, it takes us eight (8) very long years to begin mental health care for these Americans. By the time treatment does begin, the costs of mental health care services are higher and their clinical effectiveness is reduced.

That's why both the National Council and the CBHC are so excited about Mental Health First Aid. It is an evidence based practice that represents an early intervention and early detection program that --if implemented broadly enough – could permit America's community mental health providers to help millions of our fellow citizens in psychiatric distress. In brief, Mental Health First Aid teaches a diverse array of audiences three important sets of skills:

- Recognition of the signs and symptoms of common mental illnesses like bipolar disorder, major clinical depression, PTSD and anxiety disorders.
- Crisis de-escalation techniques.
- A five step action plan to get persons in psychiatric distress referred to mental health providers including local Community Mental Health Centers.

In sum, this training is somewhat similar to first aid classes taught by local chapters of the Red Cross for physical health conditions.

In our state, we receive some funding from the Colorado Office of Behavioral Health, which is the state mental health authority, and use Community Mental Health Center resources to provide Mental Health First Aid in various locations through out Colorado. People who want to attend a Mental Health First Aid class can log on to a Website, or contact their local mental health center and enroll in classes happening in their local communities. All of our Community Mental Health Centers have trained Mental Health First Aid instructors.

As I indicated at the outset, a diverse array of training audiences is key to the program's public health approach. For example, Mental Health First Aid Instructors have conducted trainings with the State Sheriff's Association and the Colorado Department of Corrections. In fact, the DOC has a goal of training all their corrections and parole officers.

The Committee might be interested to know that we've trained Governor Hickenlooper's Cabinet members, Department Heads, and the middle managers at many State agencies. CBHC is currently organizing Mental Health First Aid training for all the rabbis in the Denver Metropolitan Area. We would also like to extend the training to schools districts and institutions of higher education throughout the state. The ultimate goal is to increase the understanding of mental health issues, help our citizens be able to identify when a friend, co-worker or family member is having mental health distress, and help them get involved in treatment when it is necessary. Someday we hope to see Mental Health First Aid Instruction as common place as physical health first aid.

In all candor, the tragic movie theater shootings in Aurora, Colorado added a strong impetus to all these efforts in Colorado. Indeed, in the aftermath of the enormous tragedy at Sandy Hook Elementary School in Newtown, CT., there has an outpouring of bipartisan support for improving the mental health care system in this nation. Voices as diverse as the Wall Street Journal editorial page, the libertarian Cato Institute, President George W. Bush's former speech writer and, now, Vice President Biden's Gun Violence Task Force have all endorsed various proposals to enhance mental health care in schools and improve services for people with severe mental disorders. In fact, the task force explicitly endorsed Mental Health First Aid.

We note that there is a common policy thread running through all these proposals. In some form or fashion, they all endorse "early detection" of mental illnesses. The National Council and CBHC strongly endorse Mental Health First Aid because – from a prevention standpoint – that is exactly what the program does. It permits to us intervene early in the lives of individuals who later may be in desperate need of more intensive community-based mental health services.

Last week, Rep. Ron Barber introduced the Mental Health Aid Act of 2013 (H.R. 274). Congressman Barber was grievously wounded in the tragic Tucson, Arizona shooting the almost took the life of former-Representative Gabrielle Giffords and left six other persons dead including a 9 year old girl. We have it on good authority that Sen. Mark Begich will soon introduce the companion bill in the U.S. Senate. He will be joined by Sen. Kelly Ayotte from New Hampshire.

In a recent letter to Vice President Biden, Congressman Barber wrote the following: "I urge you to endorse common-sense, bipartisan proposals like the Mental Health First Aid Act. We have failed to give the mental health care needs of Americans Due attention for too long – and we paid too high a price for this neglect."

In the perhaps divisive legislative debate to come, we hope that the Senate HELP Committee can come together to enact the "common sense, bipartisan proposals" that Rep. Barber referred to in his correspondence the vice president.

Again, thanks for the opportunity to testify. I am happy to answer any questions you may have.

George DelGrosso,
CEO
Colorado Behavioral Healthcare Council

In: U.S. Mental Health Workforce ...
Editor: Maurice Gordon

ISBN: 978-1-62948-865-3
© 2014 Nova Science Publishers, Inc.

*Chapter 8*

# TESTIMONY OF ROBERT PETZEL, UNDER SECRETARY FOR HEALTH, VETERANS HEALTH ADMINISTRATION, DEPARTMENT OF VETERANS AFFAIRS. HEARING ON "VA MENTAL HEALTH CARE: ENSURING TIMELY ACCESS TO HIGH-QUALITY CARE"[*]

Good morning, Chairman Sanders, Ranking Member Burr and Members of the Committee. Thank you for the opportunity to discuss VA's delivery of comprehensive mental health care and services to our Nation's Veterans and their families. I am accompanied today by Dr. Sonja Batten, Deputy Chief Consultant for Specialty Mental Health; Dr. Janet Kemp, National Mental Health Program Director, Suicide Prevention and Community engagement, Mental Health Services, and Dr. William Busby, Acting Chief Officer for Readjustment Counseling Service.

Since September 11, 2001, more than two million Service members have deployed to Iraq or Afghanistan with unprecedented duration and frequency. Long deployments and intense combat conditions require optimal support for the emotional and mental health needs of our Veterans and their families. VA continues to develop and expand its mental health delivery system. VA has learned a great deal about both the strengths of our mental health care system, and the areas that need improvement.

---

[*] This is an edited, reformatted and augmented version of a testimony, presented March 20, 2013 before the Senate Committee on Veterans' Affairs.

VA is working closely with our Federal partners to implement President Barack Obama's Executive Order 13625, "Improve Access to Mental Health Services for Veterans, Service Members, and Military Families," signed on August 31, 2012. The executive order reaffirmed the President's commitment to preventing suicide, increasing access to mental health services, and supporting innovative research on relevant mental health conditions. The executive order strengthens suicide prevention efforts by increasing capacity at the Veterans/Military Crisis Line and through supporting the implementation of a national suicide prevention campaign. The executive order supports recovery-oriented mental health services for Veterans by directing the hiring of 800 peer specialists, to bring this expertise to our mental health teams. It also supports VA in using a variety of recruitment strategies to hire 1,600 new mental health clinicians and 300 administrative personnel in support of the mental health programs. Furthermore, it strengthens partnerships between VA and community providers by directing VA to work with the Department of Health and Human Services (HHS), to establish 15 pilot agreements with HHS-funded community clinics to improve access to mental health services in pilot communities, and to develop partnerships in hiring providers in rural areas. Finally, it promotes mental health research and development of more effective treatment methodologies in collaboration between VA, Department of Defense (DOD), HHS, and Department of Education.

VHA has begun work on implementing the Fiscal Year 2013 National Defense Authorization Act (P.L. 112-239) (NDAA), signed on January 2, 2013, including developing measures to assess mental health care timeliness, patient satisfaction, capacity and availability of evidence-based therapies, as well as developing staffing guidelines for specialty and general mental health. In addition, VA is developing a contract with the National Academy of Sciences to consult on the development and implementation of measures and guidelines, and to assess the quality of mental health care.

My written statement will describe VA's mental health care delivery system with specialized programs in suicide prevention, post-traumatic stress disorder (PTSD), and military sexual trauma as well as readjustment counseling. It highlights ongoing research in mental health, our process for continuous quality improvement as well as the measurement of that improvement. It also describes our outreach and access initiatives and VA's recent enhancement of mental health staffing.

VA operates one of the largest, highest-quality integrated healthcare systems. VA is a pioneer in mental health research, discovering and utilizing effective, high-quality, evidence-based treatments. It has made deployment of evidence-based therapies a critical element of its approach to mental health care. State-of-the-art treatment, including both psychotherapies and biomedical treatments, are available for the full range of mental health problems, such as PTSD, consequences of military sexual trauma, substance use disorders, and suicidality. While VA is primarily focused on evidence-based treatments, we are also assessing those complementary and alternative treatment methodologies that need further research, such as meditation and acupuncture in the care of PTSD.

VHA provides a continuum of recovery-oriented, patient-centered services across outpatient, residential, and inpatient settings. VA has trained over 4,700 VA mental health professionals to provide two of the most effective evidence-based psychotherapies for PTSD: Cognitive Processing Therapy and Prolonged Exposure Therapy. Veterans treated with these psychotherapies report fewer PTSD symptoms. The reported reduction in PTSD symptoms, an average of 19-20 points on the Post –Traumatic Stress Disorder Checklist , is clinically significant. Furthermore, VA operates the National Center for PTSD, which guides a national PTSD Mentoring program, working with every specialty PTSD program across the VA system to improve care. The Center has also begun to operate a PTSD Consultation Program open to any VA practitioner (including primary care practitioners and Homeless Program coordinators) who requests expert consultation regarding a Veteran in treatment with PTSD. So far, 500 VA practitioners have utilized this service. The Center further supports clinicians by sending subscribers updates on the latest clinically relevant trauma and PTSD research, including the Clinician's Trauma Update Online, PTSD Research Quarterly, and the PTSD Monthly Update. As IOM observed in its recent report, "Spurred by the return of large numbers of veterans from [Operation Enduring Freedom/Operation Iraqi Freedom/Operation New Dawn (OEF/OIF/OND)], the VA has substantially increased the number of services for veterans who have PTSD and worked to improve the consistency of access to such services. Every medical center and at least the largest community-based outpatient clinics are expected to have specialized PTSD services available onsite. Mental health staff members devoted to the treatment of OIF and OEF Veterans have also been deployed throughout the system."

Specialized care is available for Veterans who experienced military sexual trauma (MST) while serving on active duty or active duty for training. All sexual trauma-related care and counseling is provided free of charge to all Veterans, even if they are not eligible for other VA care. In fiscal year (FY) 2012, every VHA facility provided MST related outpatient care to both women and men, and a total of 64,161 Veterans who screened positive for MST received a total of 725,000 outpatient MST-related mental health clinical visits. This is a 13.3 percent increase from the previous year (FY 2011). Additionally, in FY 2012, of those who received care in a VA medical center or clinic, over 500,000 Veterans with a Substance Use Disorder (SUD) diagnosis received treatment for this problem. VA developed and disseminated clinical guidance to newly hired SUD-PTSD specialists who are promoting integrated care for these co-occurring conditions, and provided direct services to over 18,000 of these Veterans in FY 2012.

Use of complementary and alternative medicine (CAM) for treating mental health problems is widespread in VA. A 2011 survey of all VA facilities by VA's Healthcare Information and Analysis Group found that 89 percent of VA facilities offered CAM. VA's Office of Research and Development (ORD) recently undertook a dedicated effort to evaluate CAM in the treatment of PTSD with the solicitation of research applications examining the efficacy of meditative approaches to PTSD treatment. The result was three new clinical trials; all are currently underway, recruiting participants with PTSD. VA has also begun pilot testing a mechanism for conducting multi-site clinical CAM demonstration projects within mental health that will provide a roadmap for identifying innovative treatment methods, measuring their efficacy and effectiveness, and generating recommendations for system-wide implementation as warranted by the data. Nine medical facilities with meditation programs were selected for participation in the clinical demonstration projects. A team of subject matter experts in mind-body medicine from the University of Rochester has been asked to provide an objective, external evaluation. The majority of the clinical demonstration projects are expected to be completed this month, and the aggregate final report by the outside evaluation team is due later in 2013.

Even one Veteran suicide is too many. VA is committed to ensuring the safety of our Veterans, especially when they are in crisis. Our suicide prevention program is based on the principle that in order to decrease rates of suicide, we must provide enhanced access to high quality mental health care and develop programs specifically designed to help prevent suicide. In partnership with the Substance Abuse and Mental Health Services Administration's National Suicide Prevention Lifeline, the Veterans Crisis Line (VCL) connects Veterans in crisis and their families and friends with qualified, caring Department of Veterans Affairs responders through a confidential toll-free hotline that offers 24/7 emergency assistance. VCL has recently expanded to include a chat option and texting option for contacting the Crisis Line. Since its establishment five years ago, the VCL has made approximately 26,000 rescues of actively suicidal Veterans. The program continues to save lives and link Veterans with effective ongoing mental health services on a daily basis. In FY 2012, VCL received 193,507 calls, resulting in 6,462 rescues, any one of which may have been life-saving. In accordance with the President's August 31, 2012, Executive Order, VA has completed hiring and training of additional staff to increase the capacity of the Veterans Crisis Line by 50 percent. However, VCL is only one component of the VA overarching suicide prevention program that is based on the premise that ready access to high quality care can prevent suicide.

VA has placed Suicide Prevention Teams at each facility. The leaders of these teams, the Suicide Prevention Coordinators, are specifically devoted to preventing suicide among Veterans, and the implementation of the program at their facilities. The coordinators play a key role in VA's work to prevent suicide both in individual patients and in the entire Veteran population. Among many other functions, coordinators ensure that referrals from all sources, including the Crisis Line, e-mail, and word of mouth referrals are appropriately responded to in a timely manner. Coordinators educate their colleagues, Veterans and families about risks for suicide, coordinate staff education programs about suicide prevention, and verify that clinical providers are trained. They provide enhanced treatment monitoring for veterans at risk. They assure continued care and treatment by verifying that each "high risk" Veteran has a medical record notification entered; that they receive a suicide-specific enhanced care package, and any missed appointments are followed up on. The coordinators track and monitor all suicide-related events in an internal data collection system. This allows VA to determine trends and common risk factors, and provides information on where and how best to address concerns.

VA has developed two hubs of expertise, one at the Canandaigua Center of Excellence for Suicide Prevention (Canandaigua, NY), and another at the VISN 19 Mental Illness Research Education and Clinical Center (Denver, CO), to conduct research regarding intervention, treatments and messaging approaches and has developed a Suicide Consultation Program for practitioners that opened in 2013 and is already in use.

On February 1, 2013, VA released a report on Veteran suicides, a result of the most comprehensive review of Veteran suicide rates ever undertaken by the VA. With assistance from state partners providing real-time data, VA is now better able to assess the effectiveness of its suicide prevention programs and identify specific populations that need targeted interventions. This new information will assist VA to identify where at risk Veterans may be located and improve the Department's ability to target specific suicide interventions and outreach activities in order to reach Veterans early and proactively. The data will also help VA continue to examine the effectiveness of suicide prevention programs being implemented in specific geographic locations (e.g., rural areas), as well as care settings, such as primary care in order to replicate effective programs in other areas. VA is continuing to receive state data and will update the Suicide Data report later this year. Thus far, 39 states have reported suicide data to VA; 6 additional states are preparing data for shipment. VA reviews the data submitted by states to validate Veteran status.

In addition, VA has established the Mental Health Innovations Task Force, which is working to identify and implement early intervention strategies for specific high-risk groups. For example, Veterans with PTSD, pain, sleep disorders; depression and substance use disorders are at high risk for suicide. Through early intervention, we hope to reduce the likelihood that Veterans in these groups will progress into even higher risk status.

At VA, we have the responsibility to anticipate the needs of returning Veterans. Mental health care at VA is an extensive system of comprehensive treatments and services to meet the individual mental health needs of Veterans. We have many entry points for VHA mental health care: through our 152 medical centers, 821 community-based outpatient clinics, 300 Vet Centers that provide readjustment counseling, the Veterans Crisis Line, VA staff on college and university campuses and other outreach efforts.

Since FY 2006, the number of Veterans receiving specialized mental health treatment has risen each year, from 927,052 to more than 1.3 million in FY 2012, partly due to proactive screening to identify Veterans who may have symptoms of depression, PTSD, problematic use of alcohol, or who have experienced MST. Outpatient visits have increased from 14 million in FY 2009 to over 17 million in FY 2012. Vet Centers are another avenue for access, providing services to 193,665 Veterans and their families in FY 2012. The Vet Center Combat Call Center, an around-the-clock confidential call center where combat Veterans and their families can talk with staff, comprised of fellow combat Veterans from several eras, has handled over 37,300 calls in FY 2012. The Vet Center Combat Call Center is a peer support line, providing a complementary resource to the Veterans Crisis Line, which provides 24/7 crisis intervention services. This represents a nearly 470 percent increase from FY 2011.

In response to increased demand over the last four years, VA has enhanced its capacity to deliver needed mental health services and to improve the system of care so that services can be more readily accessed by Veterans.

VA believes that mental health care must constantly evolve and improve as new research knowledge becomes available. As more Veterans access our services, we recognize their unique needs and needs of their families—many of whom have been affected by multiple, lengthy deployments. In addition, proactive screening and an enhanced sensitivity to issues being raised by Veterans have identified areas for improvement.

For example, in August 2011, VA conducted an informal survey of line-level staff at several facilities, and learned of concerns that Veterans' ability to schedule timely appointments may not match data gathered by VA's performance management system. These providers articulated constraints on their ability to best serve Veterans, including inadequate staffing, space shortages, limited hours of operation, and competing demands for other types of appointments, particularly for compensation and pension or disability evaluations. In response to this finding, VA took three major actions. First, VA developed a comprehensive action plan aimed at overcoming barriers to access, and addressing the concerns raised by its staff in the survey as well as concerns raised by Veterans and Veterans groups. Second, VA conducted focus groups with Veterans and VA staff, conducted through a contract with Altarum, to better understand the issues raised by front-line providers. Third, VA conducted a comprehensive first-hand assessment of the mental health program at every VA medical center and is working within its facilities and Veterans Integrated Service Networks (VISNs) to improve mental health programs and share best practices.

Ensuring access to appropriate care is essential to helping Veterans recover from the injuries or illnesses they incurred during their military service. Access can be realized in many ways and through many modalities, including:

- through face-to-face visits;
- telehealth;
- phone calls;
- online systems;
- mobile apps and technology;
- readjustment counseling;
- outreach;
- community partnerships; and
- academic affiliations.

In an effort to increase access to mental health care and reduce the stigma of seeking such care, VA has integrated mental health into primary care settings. The ongoing transfer of VA primary care to Patient Aligned Care Teams will facilitate the delivery of an unprecedented level of mental health services. As the recent IOM report on Treatment for Posttraumatic Stress Disorder in Military and Veteran Populations noted, it is VA policy to screen every patient seen in primary care in VA medical settings for PTSD, MST, depression, and problem drinking. The screening takes place during a patient's first appointment, and screenings for depression and problem drinking are repeated annually for as long as the Veteran uses VA services. Furthermore, PTSD screening is repeated annually for the first 5 years after the most recent separation from service and every 5 years thereafter. Systematic screening of Veterans for conditions such as depression, PTSD, problem drinking, and MST has helped VA identify more Veterans at risk for these conditions and provided opportunities to refer them to specially trained experts. The PTSD screening tool used by VA has been shown to have high levels of sensitivity and specificity.

Since the start of FY 2008, VA has provided more than 2.5 million Primary Care-Mental Health Integration (PC-MHI) clinical visits to more than 700,000 unique Veterans. This improves both access by bringing care closer to where the Veteran can most easily receive these services, and quality of care by increasing the coordination of all aspects of care, both physical and mental. Among primary care patients with positive screens for depression, those who receive same-day PC-MHI services are more than twice as likely to receive depression treatment than those who did not. Treatment works and there is hope for recovery for Veterans who need mental health care. These are important advances, particularly given the rising numbers of Veterans seeking mental health care.

VA offers expanded access to mental health services with longer clinic hours, telemental health capability to deliver services, and standards that mandate rapid access to mental health services. Telemental health allows VA to leverage technology to provide Veterans quicker and more efficient access to mental health care by reducing the distance they have to travel, increasing the flexibility of the system they use, and improving their overall quality of life. This technology improves access to general and specialty services in geographically remote areas where it can be difficult to recruit mental health professionals. Currently, the clinic-based telehealth program involves the more than 580 VA community-based outpatient clinics (CBOCs) where many Veterans receive primary care. In areas where the CBOCs do not have a mental health care provider available, VA is implementing a new program to use secure video teleconferencing technology to connect the Veteran to a provider within VA's nationwide system of care. Further, the program is expanding directly into the home of the Veteran with VA's goal to connect approximately 2,000 patients by the end of FY2013 using Internet Protocol (IP) video on Veterans' personal computers.

VA has made good progress towards providing all of those in need with evidence-based treatments, and we are now working to optimize the delivery of these tools by using novel technologies. From delivery of the treatments to rural Veterans in their homes, to supporting treatment protocols with mobile apps, VA's objective is to consistently deliver the highest quality mental health care to Veterans wherever they are. The multi-award winning PTSD Coach, co-developed with the DOD, has been downloaded nearly 100,000 times in 74 countries since mid-2011. It is being adapted by government agencies and non-profit organizations in 7 other countries including Canada and Australia. This app is notable as it aims to assist Veterans with recognizing and managing PTSD symptoms, whether or not they are comfortable engaging with VA mental health care.

For those who are kept from needed care because of logistics or fear of stigma, PTSD Coach provides an opportunity to better understand and manage the symptoms associated with PTSD as a first step toward recovery. For those who are working with VA providers, whether in specialty clinics or primary care, this app provides evidence-informed tools for self-management and symptom tracking between sessions. VA is planning to shortly roll out a version of this app that is connected to the electronic health record for active VA patients.

A wide array of mobile applications to support the evidence-based mental and behavioral health care of Veterans will be rolled out over the course of 2013. These apps are intended to be used in the context of clinical care with trained professionals and are based on gold-standard protocols for addressing smoking cessation, PTSD and suicidality.

Apps for self-management of the consequences of traumatic brain injury and crisis management, some of the more challenging issues facing Veterans and our healthcare system, will follow later in the year. Mobile apps can help Veterans build resilience and manage day-to-day challenges even in the absence of mental health disorders. Working with DOD, VA will release mobile apps for problem-solving and parenting in 2013 to help Veterans navigate common post-deployment challenges. Because we understand that healthy families are at the center of a healthy life, we are creating tools for families and caregivers of Veterans as well, including the PTSD Family Coach, a mobile app geared towards friends and families that is expected to be rolled out in mid-2013.

Technology allows us to extend our reach, not just beyond the clinic walls but to those who need help but have not yet sought our services, and to those who care for them and support their personal and professional missions. In November 2012, VA and DoD launched www.startmovingforward.org, interactive Web-based educational life-coaching program based on the principles of Problem Solving Therapy. It allows for anonymous, self-paced, 24-hour-a-day access that can be used independently or in conjunction with mental health treatment.

VA's Readjustment Counseling Service (RCS) provides a range of readjustment counseling services to those who have served in combat zones and their families. In addition to the integration of mental health with primary care, VA also provides comprehensive readjustment counseling for Veterans who have experienced military sexual trauma, as well as, bereavement counseling to families whose Servicemember died while on active duty. These services are provided in a safe and confidential environment through a National network of 300 community-based Vet Centers located in all 50 states, the District of Columbia, American Samoa, Guam, and Puerto Rico, 70 Mobile Vet Centers, and the Vet Center Combat Call Center. In FY 2012, through Vet Centers, RCS provided over 1.5 million visits to Veterans and their families, a 9 percent increase in visits from FY 2011. The Vet Center program has cumulatively provided services to 458,795 OEF/OIF/OND Veterans and their families. This represents over 30 percent of the OEF/OIF/OND Veterans who have left active duty. Furthermore, in FY 2012, Vet Center staff provided over 21,000 unique families with over 117,500 visits to help aid in the readjustment of their Veterans. This represents a 15 percent increase in the number of families and 28 percent increase in the number of visits when compared to the previous fiscal year. The increase in services provided to families is a direct result of the Secretary of Veterans Affairs Initiative to place a licensed and qualified family counselor at every Vet Center.

A core component of the Vet Center mission is to help those who served and their families overcome barriers they may have to accessing VA care and services. This is accomplished through an extensive program of face-to-face community outreach. Since the onset of the program in 1979, Vet Center staff have actively engaged their fellow Veterans and family members at targeted community events and provided them with access to services. Recently, RCS has enhanced its outreach capacity to recently returning combat Veterans through a fleet of 70 Mobile Vet Centers (MVC). To ensure early intervention and access to services the MVCs provide outreach and onsite confidential readjustment counseling to Veterans who are geographically distant from existing Vet Centers. RCS also offers services through the Vet Center Combat Call Center (877-WAR-VETS), an around the clock confidential call center where those that served in combat zone and their families can call and talk about their military service and transition home. The call center is staffed by combat Veterans from different eras as well as family members of combat Veterans.

In 2010, Public Law 111-163 expanded eligibility of Vet Center services to members of the Armed Forces (and their family members), including members of the National Guard or Reserve, who served on active duty in the Armed Forces in OEF/OIF/OND. VA and DOD are finalizing the regulatory process outlined in the law and are working together to implement this expansion of services. The recently passed FY 2013 NDAA also includes provisions that expand Vet Center eligibility to members of the Armed Forces who served in any theater of combat and to certain members of the Armed Forces, Veterans, and their family members indirectly exposed to the trauma of war. One cornerstone of the Vet Center program's success is the added level of confidentiality for Veterans and their families. Vet Centers maintain a separate system of records, which affords the confidentiality vital to serving a combat-exposed warrior population. Without the Veteran's voluntary signed authorization, the Vet Centers will not disclose Veteran clients' information unless required by law. Early access to readjustment counseling in a safe and confidential setting has proven an effective way to reduce the risk of suicide and promote the recovery of Servicemembers returning from combat. Furthermore, more than 72 percent of all Vet Center staff members are Veterans themselves. This allows the Vet Center staff to make an early empathic connection with Veterans who might not otherwise seek services even if they are much needed.

In November 2011, VA launched an award-winning, national public awareness campaign, Make the Connection, aimed at reducing the stigma associated with seeking mental health care and informing Veterans, their families, friends, and members of their communities about VA resources (www.maketheconnection.net). The candid Veteran videos on the Web site have been viewed over 4 million times, and over 1.5 million individuals have "liked" the Facebook page for the campaign (www.facebook.com/VeteransMTC). AboutFace, launched in May 2012, is a complementary public awareness campaign created by the National Center for PTSD (www.ptsd.va.gov/public/about_face.html). This initiative aims to help Veterans recognize whether the problems they are dealing with may be PTSD related and to make them aware that effective treatment can help them "turn their lives around." The National Center for PTSD has been using social media to reach out to Veterans utilizing both Facebook and Twitter. In FY 2012, there were 18,000 Facebook "fans" (up from 1,800 in 2011), making 16 posts per month and almost 7,000 Twitter followers (up from 1,700 in 2011) with 20 "tweets" per month. The PTSD Web site, www.ptsd.va.gov, received 2.3 million visits during FY2012.

VA, in collaboration with DOD, continues to focus on suicide prevention though its year-long public awareness campaign, "Stand By Them," which encourages family members and friends of Veterans to know the signs of crisis and encourage Veterans to seek help, or to reach out themselves on behalf of the Veteran using online services on www.veteranscrisisline.net. VA's current suicide awareness and education Public Service Announcement titled "Common Journey" has been running in the top one percent of the PSA Nielsen ratings since before the holidays. It is now being replaced with a PSA designed specifically to augment the Stand By Them Campaign titled "Side By Side," which was launched nationally in January 2013.

In order to further serve family members who are concerned about a Veteran, VA has expanded the "Coaching Into Care" call line nationally after a successful pilot in two VISNs. Since the inception of the service January 2010 through November 2012, "Coaching Into Care" has logged 5,154 total calls and contacts. Seventy percent of the callers are female, and most callers are spouses or family members. On 49 percent of the calls, the target is a Veteran of OEF/OIF/OND conflicts; Vietnam or immediately post-Vietnam era Veterans comprises the next highest portion (27 percent).

VA recently developed and released a "Community Provider Toolkit" which is an on-line resource for community mental health providers to learn more about mental health needs and treatments for Veterans. The Veterans Crisis Line has approximately 50 Memoranda of Agreement with community and internal VA organizations to refer callers, accept calls, and provide and receive services for callers. Furthermore, suicide Prevention Coordinators at each VA facility are required to provide a minimum of 5 outreach activities a month to their communities to increase awareness of suicide and promote community involvement in the area of Veteran suicide prevention.

VA has been working closely with outside resources to address gaps and create a more patient-centric network of care focused on wellness-based outcomes. In response to the Executive Order, VA is working closely with HHS to establish 15 pilot projects with community-based providers, such as community mental health clinics, community health centers, substance abuse treatment facilities, and rural health clinics, to test the effectiveness of community partnerships in helping to meet the mental health needs of Veterans in a timely way.

VA will continue to work closely with DOD to educate Servicemembers, VA staff, Veterans and their families, public officials, Veterans Service Organizations, and other stakeholders about all mental health resources that are available in VA and with other community partners. VA has partnered with DOD to develop the VA/DOD Integrated Mental Health Strategy (IMHS) to advance a coordinated public health model to improve access, quality, effectiveness and efficiency of mental health services for Service members, National Guard and Reserve, Veterans, and their families.

VA is committed to hiring and utilizing more mental health professionals to improve access to mental health care for Veterans. Access enables VHA to provide personalized, proactive, patient-driven health care; achieve measurable improvements in health outcomes, and align resources to deliver sustained value to Veterans.

To serve the growing number of Veterans seeking mental health care, VA has deployed significant resources and is increasing the number of staff in support of mental health services. VA has taken aggressive action to recruit, hire, and retain mental health professionals to improve Veterans' access to mental health care. VHA has made significant progress to this end, by hiring a total of 3,354 clinical and administrative support staff to directly serve Veterans since May 2012. This progress has improved the Department's ability to provide timely, quality mental health care for Veterans.

As a result, VA is able to serve Veterans better by providing enhanced services, expanded access, longer clinic hours, and increased telemental health capability to deliver services.

In FY 2012, the Office of Mental Health Operations (OMHO) conducted site visits at all 140 VHA Healthcare Systems. The site visits reviewed the implementation of the Uniform Mental Health Services Handbook (UMHSII) and involved meetings with facility leadership; mental health leadership; mental health program leadership; front-line staff, including clerks and schedulers; Veterans who receive mental health care and their families or supportive others; and community stakeholders and partners. In addition to interview data obtained in the 2 day visit, administrative data was reviewed for each healthcare system, including: Mental Health Information System data, relevant reports provided by the facility (e.g., The Joint Commission, System-wide Ongoing Assessment and Review Strategy, Commission on Accreditation of Rehabilitation Facilities, etc.), and other data obtained from multiple sources across VHA (e.g., Office of Productivity, Efficiency and Staffing, Allocation Resource Center, Mental Health Services, etc.).

- Areas identified for systemic improvement included:
- Ensuring adequate Mental Health staff;
- Improving the timeliness of Mental Health services;
- Improving scheduling of Mental Health services; and
- Increasing provision of required Mental Health services at Community-Based Outpatient Clinics (CBOC).
- Areas that were identified as for systemic improvement and also identified as systemic strengths included:
- Integration of mental health services into Primary Care;
- Care coordination across levels of care;
- Implementations of evidence-based treatments; and
- Implementation of recovery-oriented care.
- Areas identified as systemic strengths included:
- Suicide prevention services; and
- Development of diverse community partnerships.

Systemic actions that have resulted from the visits include

- The use of targeted facilitation processes for programs at VHA healthcare systems which may experience challenges in implementation, including Primary Care-Mental Health Integration and evidence-based psychotherapy;
- Continued monitoring of Mental Health staffing levels, access and scheduling, in conjunction with education and support for new wait time metrics;
- Expansion of telehealth services to outlying CBOCs and in the home; and
- Expanded dissemination of Strong Practices SharePoint for Mental Health to support cross facility learning.

In addition, VHA healthcare systems are implementing site specific action plans in response to recommendations from each facility site visit. These plans are monitored quarterly. OMHO will be visiting approximately 1/3 of VHA healthcare systems each year (45 in FY 2013) from FY 2013 forward to review continued implementation of the UMHSH, visiting each facility once every 3 years.

VHA began collecting monthly vacancy data in January 2012 to assess the impact of vacancies on operations and to develop recommendations for further improvement. In addition, VA is ensuring that accurate projections for future needs for mental health services are generated. Finally, VA is planning proactively for the expected needs of Veterans who will soon separate from active duty status as they return from Afghanistan.

Since there are no industry standards defining accurate mental health staffing ratios, VHA is setting the standard, as we have for other dimensions of mental health care. VHA has developed a prototype staffing model for general mental health delivery and is expanding the model to include specialty mental health care. VHA developed and implemented an aggressive recruitment and marketing effort to fill existing vacancies in mental health care occupations. To support implementation of the guidance, VHA announced the hiring of 1,600 new mental health professionals and 300 support staff in April 2012. Key initiatives include targeted advertising and outreach, aggressive recruitment from a pipeline of qualified trainees/residents to leverage against mission critical mental health vacancies, and providing consultative services to VISN and VA stakeholders. Despite the national challenges with recruitment of mental health care professionals, VHA continues to make significant improvements in its recruitment and retention efforts. Focused efforts are underway to expand the pool of applicants for those professions and sites where hiring is most difficult, such as creating expanded mental health training programs in rural areas and through recruitment and retention incentives.

As part of our ongoing comprehensive review of mental health operations, VHA has considered a number of factors to determine additional staffing levels distributed across the system, including:

- Veteran population in the service area;
- The mental health needs of Veterans in that population; and
- Range and complexity of mental health services provided in the service area.

Specialty mental health care occupations, such as psychologists, psychiatrists, and others, are difficult to fill and will require a very aggressive recruitment and marketing effort. VHA has developed a strategy for this effort focusing on the following key factors:

- Implementing a highly visible, multi-faceted, and sustained marketing and outreach campaign targeted to mental health care providers;
- Engaging VHA's National Health Care Recruiters for the most difficult to recruit positions;
- Recruiting from an active pipeline of qualified candidates to leverage against vacancies; and
- Ensuring complete involvement and support from VA leadership.

VA is committed to hiring and utilizing more mental health professionals to improve access to mental health care for Veterans. To serve the growing number of Veterans seeking mental health care, VA has deployed significant resources and is increasing the number of staff in support of mental health services. VA has taken aggressive action to recruit, hire, and retain mental health professionals to improve Veterans' access to mental health care. The department also has used many tools to hire the mental health workforce, including pay-setting authorities, loan repayment, scholarship programs and partnerships with health care workforce training programs to recruit and retain one of the largest mental health care workforces in the Nation. As a result, VA is able to serve Veterans better by providing enhanced services, expanded access, longer clinic hours, and increased telemental health capability to deliver services.

In April 2012, VA announced a goal to hire an additional 1,600 clinical providers and 300 administrative support staff. As of March 5, 2013, VA has hired 1,089 clinical providers and 230 administrative staff in support of this specific goal. President Obama's August 31, 2012, executive order requires the positions to be filled by June 30, 2013.

VA is strategically working with universities, colleges and health professional training institutions across the country to expand their curricula to address the new science related to meeting the mental and behavioral needs of our Nation's Veterans, Servicemembers, Wounded Warriors, and their family members. In addition to ongoing job placement and outreach efforts through VetSuccess, VA has implemented a new outreach program, "Veterans Integration to Academic Leadership," that places VA mental health staff at 21 colleges and universities to work with Veterans attending school on the GI Bill.

VA's Office of Academic Affiliations trains roughly 6,400 trainees in mental health occupations per year (including 3,400 in psychiatry, 1,900 in psychology, and 1,100 in social work, plus clinical pastoral education positions). Currently, VA has one of only two accredited psychology internship programs in the entire state of Alaska. VA is committed to expanding training opportunities in mental health professions in order to build a pipeline of future VA health care providers. VA continues to expand mental health training opportunities in Nursing, Pharmacy, Psychiatry, Psychology, and Social Work. For example, over 202 positions were approved to begin in academic year 2013-2014 at 43 VHA facilities focused on the expansion of existing accredited programs in integrated care settings such as General Outpatient Mental Health Clinics or Patient Aligned Care Teams (PACT). These include over 86 training positions for Outpatient Mental Health Interprofessional Teams and 116 training positions for PACTs with Mental Health Integration, specifically 12 positions in Nursing, 43 in Pharmacy, over 34 in Psychiatry, 62 in Psychology, and 51 in Social Work. The Office of Academic Affiliations is scheduled to release the Phase II Mental Health Training Expansion Request for Proposals in Spring 2013 which will further assist with VA future workforce needs.

There are many Veterans who are willing to seek treatment and to share their experiences with mental health issues when they share a common bond of duty, honor, and service with the provider. While providing evidence-based psychotherapies is critical, VA understands Veterans benefit from supportive services other Veterans can provide. To meet this need in accordance with the Executive Order and as part of VA's efforts to implement section 304 of Public Law 111-163 (Caregivers and Veterans Omnibus Health Services Act of 2010), VA has hired over 140 Peer Specialists and Apprentices in recent months, and is hiring and training nearly 660 more. Additionally, VA has awarded a contract to the Depression and Bipolar Support Alliance to provide certification training for Peer Specialists. This peer staff is expected to be hired by December 31, 2013, and will work as members of mental health teams. Simultaneously, VA is providing additional resources to expand peer support services across the Nation to support full-time, paid peer support technicians.

VA is reengineering its performance measurement methodologies to evaluate and revamp its programs. Performance measurement and accountability will remain the cornerstones of our program to ensure that resources are being devoted where they need to go and are being used to the benefit of Veterans. Our priority is leading the Nation in patient satisfaction regarding the quality, effectiveness of care and timeliness of their appointments.

Recognizing the benefit that would come from improving Veteran access, VA is modifying the current appointment performance measurement system to include a combination of measures that better captures each Veteran's needs. VA will ensure this approach is structured around a thoughtful, individualized treatment plan developed for each Veteran to inform the timing of appointments.

In April 2012, VA's Office of Inspector General (OIG) report on VA's mental health programs gave four recommendations: 1) a need for improvement in our wait time measurements, 2) improvement in patient experience metrics, 3) development of a staffing model, and 4) provision of data to improve clinic management. Further, in January 2013, the U.S. Government Accountability Office reviewed VA's healthcare outpatient medical appointment scheduling and appointment notification processes, specifically focusing on Veterans wait times, local VA Medical Center implementation of national scheduling policies and processes as well as VHA initiatives to improve Veterans' access to medical appointments.

In direct response, VA is using OIG and GAO results along with our internal reviews to implement important enhancements to VA mental health care. Based on OIG and GAO findings, VA is updating scheduling practices, and strengthening performance measures to ensure accountability. VA has examined how best to measure Veterans' wait time experiences and how to improve scheduling processes to define how our facilities should respond to Veterans' needs and commissioned a study to measure the association between various measures of appointment timeliness and the resulting patient satisfaction. Based on the results of this study, VA is changing its timeliness measures to best track different populations (new vs. established patients) using the approach which best predicts patient satisfaction and clinical care outcomes. The study showed that new and established patients have different needs and require different approaches for capturing wait times. The data identified that the Create Date, the date that an appointment is made, is the optimal method for new patients, since most new patients want their visit or clinical evaluation to occur as close to the time they make the appointment as possible. For established patients, VHA has determined that using the Desired Date is the most reliable and patient-centered approach. Desired Date is the ideal time a patient or provider wants the patient to be seen. Armed with evidence that the Create Date and the Desired Date best predict patient satisfaction and health outcomes for new and established patients respectively, VHA adopted these methods on October 1, 2012. With the recent evidence from our wait time study, ongoing VHA performance measures, as well as findings and recommendation from oversight entities, VHA believes it now has reliable and valid wait time measures that allow VHA to accurately measure how long a patient waits for an outpatient appointment. In addition, VA is developing measures based on timeliness after referral to mental health services, patient perceptions of barriers to care, and measures of clinic capacity. VHA's action plan is aimed at ensuring the integrity of wait time measurement data so that VHA has the most reliable information to ensure Veterans have timely access to care and high satisfaction.

VHA provides Veterans with personalized, proactive mental health care to optimize their health and well-being. The ultimate unit of outcome is the improvement in the quality of life for each Veteran. As part of its commitment to transparency, stewardship, and exceptional health care services, VHA is also eager to have a set of outcome metrics to evaluate its mental health care system. There is no national standard for measuring outcomes in mental health care. The literature indicates the best approach is to use a variety of measures including patient satisfaction, clinical quality effectiveness, and clinical process assessment. In 2011, the National Quality Forum (NQF) published a consensus report outlining a framework for mental health and substance use outcome measures. VHA has chartered a workgroup to identify a set of population-based, outcome-oriented metrics. The development and use of these measures will be an iterative process over a period of months and years, and additional metrics will be developed using additional data sources. At present, VA has selected five initial metrics, including standardized mortality ration, rates of suicide re-attempt, drug screening of patients on opioid therapy, antipsychotic medication adherence among patients with schizophrenia, and flu vaccination rates in VA mental health patients.

In 2011, VHA raised the bar for the industry by setting a wait time goal of 14 days for both primary and specialty care appointments. Last year, VHA added a goal of completing primary care appointments within 7 days of the Desired Date. The intent is to come as close as possible to providing just-in-time mental health care for patients. The ultimate goal is same day access. VHA is focused on implementing new wait time measurement practices, policies, and technologies along with aggressive monitoring of reliability through oversight and audits. By taking these steps, we are confident that we will be able to deliver accessible, high quality, timely mental health care to Veterans. The development of improved performance metrics, more reliable reporting tools, and an initial mental health staffing model, will enable VHA to better track wait times, assess productivity, and determine capacity for mental health services. All of these tools will continue to be evaluated and improved with experience in their use.

Mr. Chairman, we know our work to improve the delivery of mental health care to Veterans will never be truly finished. However, we are confident that we are building a more accessible system that will be responsive to the needs of our Veterans while being responsible with the resources appropriated by Congress. We appreciate your support and encouragement in identifying and resolving challenges as we find new ways to care for Veterans. VA is committed to providing the high quality of care that our Veterans have earned and deserve, and we continue to take every available action to improve access to mental health care services. We appreciate the opportunity to appear before you today, and my colleagues and I are prepared to respond to any questions you may have.

**Chapter 9**

# STATEMENT OF PAMELA S. HYDE, ADMINISTRATOR, SUBSTANCE ABUSE AND MENTAL HEALTH SERVICES ADMINISTRATION. HEARING ON "EXAMINING SAMHSA'S ROLE IN DELIVERING SERVICES TO THE SEVERELY MENTALLY ILL"[*]

Good morning Chairman Murphy, Ranking Member DeGette and Members of the Subcommittee.

Thank you for the opportunity to testify today about the mission and priorities of the Substance Abuse and Mental Health Services Administration (SAMHSA), including services for adults with serious mental illness and children with serious emotional disturbance. SAMHSA accomplishes its mission through partnerships, policies, products, and programs that build resilience, improve treatment, and facilitate recovery for people with or at risk for mental and substance use disorders.

---

[*] This is an edited, reformatted and augmented version of a statement presented May 22, 2013 before the House Energy & Commerce Committee, Oversight and Investigations Subcommittee.

## SAMHSA's ROLE

SAMHSA was established in 1992 and is directed by Congress to effectively target substance abuse and mental health services to the people most in need of them and to translate research in these areas more effectively and more rapidly into the general health care system. SAMHSA's mission is to reduce the impact of substance abuse and mental illness on America's communities. SAMHSA strives to create awareness that:

- Behavioral Health is essential for health;
- Prevention works;
- Treatment is effective; and
- People recover from mental and substance use disorders.

SAMHSA serves as a national voice on mental health and mental illness, substance abuse, and behavioral health systems of care. It coordinates behavioral health surveillance to better understand the impact of substance abuse and mental illness on children, individuals, and families as well as the costs associated with treatment. SAMHSA helps to ensure dollars are invested in evidence-based and data-driven programs and initiatives that result in improved health and resilience.

SAMHSA applies strategic, data-driven solutions to field-driven priorities. To this end, SAMHSA helps states, territories, and tribes build and improve basic and proven practices and system capacity by encouraging innovation, supporting more efficient approaches, and incorporating research-based programs and best practices into funded programs so they can produce measureable results. In addition, SAMHSA's longstanding partnerships with other Federal agencies, systems, national stakeholders, and the public have uniquely positioned SAMHSA to collaborate and coordinate across multiple program areas, collect best practices and develop expertise around behavioral health services, and, understand and respond to the full breadth of the behavioral health needs of children, individuals and families across the country.

Substance abuse, addictions, poor emotional health, and mental illnesses take a toll on individuals, families, and communities. These conditions cost lives and productivity, and strain families and resources in the same way as untreated as physical illnesses. SAMHSA works to focus the Nation's attention on these preventable and treatable problems.

## Mental Health and Substance Abuse Data

Health surveillance is critical to SAMHSA's ability to develop new models of care to address substance abuse and mental illness. SAMHSA provides decision makers, researchers and the general public with enhanced information about the extent of substance abuse and mental illness, how systems of care are organized and financed, when and how to seek help, and about effective models of care, including the outcomes of treatment engagement and recovery.

It is estimated that almost half of all Americans will experience symptoms of a mental health condition – mental illness or addiction – at some point in their lives. Yet, today, less than one in five children and adolescents with diagnosable mental health problems receive the treatment they need.[1] And according to data from SAMHSA's National Survey on Drug Use and Health (NSDUH), only 38% of adults with diagnosable mental health problems – and only 11% of those with diagnosable substance use disorders - receive needed treatment.[2]

With respect to the onset of behavioral health conditions, half of all lifetime cases of mental and substance use disorders begin by age 14 and three-fourths by age 24.[3]

Currently, SAMHSA supports national surveys and surveillance, including the National Survey on Drug Use and Health, Drug Abuse Warning Network, and Drug and Alcohol Service Information System. SAMHSA also supports the behavioral health field by sharing information about evidence-based practices through tools such as the National Registry of Evidence-based Programs and Practices. SAMHSA also uses the Web, print, social media, public appearances, and the press to reach the public, providers and other stakeholders, including people in recovery and their families.

## Practice Improvement

SAMHSA supports innovation and practice improvement by disseminating key evidence-based mental health and substance use practices, such as Treatment Improvement Protocols, Technical Assistance Publications, The National Registry of Evidence-based Programs and Practices, and evidenced-based toolkits, to the mental health and substance abuse delivery system and facilitates practice improvement by engaging in activities that support mental health system transformation and reform. One of SAMHSA's roles is to provide grants and contracts consistent with congressionally-appropriated funding. SAMHSA uses this crucial funding to create, test, and disseminate models of services and programs to improve the Nation's behavioral healthcare delivery systems as well as the promotion of mental health and the prevention of mental illness and addictions in children and adults. Additionally, SAMHSA holds policy academies for states, tribes and territories, provides technical assistance, training, and guidance for the behavioral health field, supports innovation in evaluation and research, moves innovations and evidence-based approaches to scale, identifies and disseminates new and emerging practices from the field, and cooperates with national and international partners to identify promising approaches to supporting behavioral health.

## Public Education and Awareness

Today in the United States, opportunities to prevent or intervene early to reduce disability and death associated with mental illness and substance use disorders are often missed. The tragedy at Sandy Hook Elementary School in December 2012 underscores the importance of educating the American people about mental health and what we can do to connect people in need with services.

By learning to recognize the signs and symptoms of mental illness and substance abuse, friends and family members can help their loved ones take action and seek care. Trained health professionals can also work with individuals and families to identify problems early.

To help with its public education effort, SAMHSA supports public awareness campaigns, produces and distributes public education materials, releases data from its surveillance and data collection efforts, and increasingly uses electronic and social media to help disseminate information to the public and the field.

By confronting fear and misunderstanding with facts, raising awareness about the effectiveness of prevention and treatment, and improving knowledge about when and where to seek help, SAMHSA helps bring mental illness and addictions out of the shadows and helps the nation achieve the full potential of the science behind the prevention and treatment of mental illnesses and substance abuse.

## Policy Development and Oversight

SAMHSA protects and promotes behavioral health through regulation and standard setting. For example, SAMHSA works to prevent tobacco sales to minors through the Synar Program, administers the Federal drug-free workplace and drug-testing programs, oversees opioid treatment programs and accreditation bodies, informs physicians' office-based opioid treatment prescribing practices, and partners with other agencies at the U.S. Department of Health and Human Services in development and review of regulations and guidance documents affecting prevention, treatment and recovery support services that address mental health and substance abuse.

## OVERVIEW OF THE NATION'S MENTAL HEALTH SPENDING

According to SAMHSA's *National Expenditures for Mental Health Services & Substance Abuse Treatment 1986 – 2009,* at $147 billion, mental health spending accounted for 6.3 percent of all health spending in calendar year 2009, while substance abuse spending accounted for approximately one percent. Mental health treatment spending depended more on public payers than spending for all-health care in calendar year 2009; public payers accounted for 60 percent of mental health spending compared to 49 percent of all-health care spending.

Medicaid and Medicare (40 percent) and private insurance (26 percent) accounted for approximately two-thirds of mental health spending in 2009, followed by state and local governments at 15 percent, out-of-pocket at 11 percent, other Federal spending at five percent (including SAMHSA funding), and other private sources at three percent.

### SAMHSA's Budget

In FY 2013, approximately 29 percent ($957.7 million) of SAMHSA's funding was appropriated or designated for mental health programs and activities, with the remainder directed to substance abuse programs and activities. This distribution of funding between substance abuse and mental health has been consistent for the last five years.

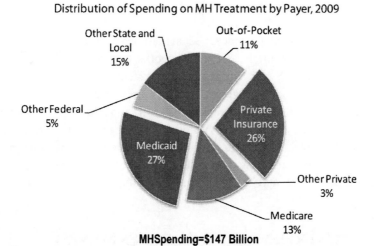

Distribution of Spending on MH Treatment by Payer, 2009

MHSpending=$147 Billion

Of the SAMHSA mental health funding, most ($915.3 million) supports prevention, treatment and recovery support programs and activities within SAMHSA's Center for Mental Health Services (CMHS). In addition to the CMHS funding, a portion ($42.4 million) of SAMHSA's funding for the Health Surveillance and Program Support (HSPS) programs is used for the mental health activities.

## Center for Mental Health Services (CMHS)

Approximately 48 percent ($436.81 million) of CMHS funding is directed toward the Community Mental Health Services Block Grant, which provides services and supports for adults with serious mental illness[4] and children with serious emotional disturbance.[5]

The balance of the CMHS budget (52 percent) provides support for a range of mental health prevention, treatment and recovery support services as directed by Congress. In FY 2013, approximately 81 percent of the CMHS budget will support adults with and at risk for serious mental illness and/or children with serious emotional disturbance.

Within the CMHS budget over the last five years, 75-80 percent of appropriated funding has been used for mental health programs in support of adults with serious mental illness and children with serious emotional disturbance.

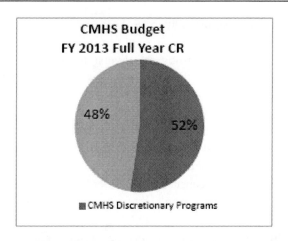

# EXAMPLES OF SAMHSA PROGRAMS WITH NATIONAL IMPACT

To accomplish its work, SAMHSA administers a combination of competitive discretionary programs and block grant programs. This portfolio provides states and communities with support to establish or expand organized community-based systems of care for children with serious emotional disturbances and adults with serious mental illness through training, technical assistance, and provision of evidenced-based clinical and recovery support services.

## Community Mental Health Services Block Grant

The Community Mental Health Services Block Grant is a key source of funding for community-based services for adults with serious mental illness and children with serious emotional disturbances. In Fiscal Year (FY) 2013, $408.9 million, was awarded to states through the Community Mental Health Services Block Grant. It is a flexible funding source used by states to provide a range of mental health services and system infrastructure and capacity supports. States use these limited but significant funds to support planning, administration, evaluation, educational activities, and direct service delivery. Services typically are for those not covered by Medicaid, insurance or other sources, and for services not otherwise covered, and include rehabilitation services, crisis stabilization and case management, peer specialist and consumer-directed services, wrap around services for children and families, supported employment and housing, jail diversion programs, and services for special populations. By law, states are not allowed to utilize these funds for inpatient services.

Each state's Community Mental Health Services Block Grant application is based on a plan developed in collaboration with state mental health planning councils, which are required in order to receive block grant funding. Planning councils' membership is statutorily mandated to include consumers, family members of adult and child consumers, providers, and representatives of other principal state agencies delivering, paying for, or impacting mental health services.

The Community Mental Health Services Block Grant supports services and infrastructure for state mental health authorities that serve almost seven million adults with serious mental illness and children with serious emotional disturbance.

SAMHSA has placed a strong emphasis on ensuring that Block Grant funds are expended in a manner consistent with the statutory and regulatory framework, including providing states the flexibility to address service needs and approaches they believe are most critical for the populations of adults with serious mental illness and children with serious emotional disturbances. Currently, the primary goals of SAMHSA program integrity efforts are to: (1) promote the proper expenditure of Block Grant funds; (2) improve Block Grant program compliance nationally; and (3) demonstrate the effective use of Block Grant funds, including using National Outcomes Measures such as readmission to any state psychiatric hospital within 30 days and 180 days; proved functioning; and employment status.

## Children's Mental Health Initiative

The Children's Mental Health Initiative (CMHI) provides $111.4 million in FY 2013 to states and communities to support the development of comprehensive, community-based systems of care for the estimated nine to 13 percent of children and youth with SED and their families. A system of care is a strategic approach to the delivery of services and supports that incorporate family-driven, youth-guided, strength-based, and culturally and linguistically competent care in order to meet the physical, intellectual, emotional, cultural, and social needs of children and youth.

CMHI has served over 120,000 children and youth with serious emotional disturbance since the inception of the program. Data from the CMHI National Evaluation demonstrates that the system-of-care approach is effective. For example, school attendance and performance improves, behavioral and emotional strengths are increased, and children and youth have more stable living conditions. Within six months of service in CMHI, the number of youth reporting suicide attempts or thoughts of suicide decreased. And, there were decreased contacts with law enforcement. Specifically, for youth involved in the juvenile justice system, arrests decreased by nearly 50 percent from intake into the program after 12 months of service in CMHI.

## The National Child Traumatic Stress Network

Through the National Child Traumatic Stress Initiative (NCTSI), SAMHSA supports a national network of grantees—the National Child Traumatic Stress Network (NCTSN)—that works collaboratively to develop and promote effective trauma treatment, services and other resources for children and adolescents exposed to an array of traumatic events. The NCTSN Centers collaborate to develop, implement, and evaluate effective trauma screening, treatment and services, and partner with other community agencies to promote service delivery approaches so that trauma services are effectively implemented within local child-serving community service systems. To date, NCTSI has developed and implemented 20 effective interventions to reduce immediate distress from exposure to traumatic events, developed and provided training in trauma-focused services for use in child mental health clinics, schools, child welfare and protective services, among other service areas; and developed widely used intervention protocols for disaster victims. In FY 2012, 2,367 children and adolescents received trauma-informed services through the NCTSI program, and over 121,310 people were trained in annual training education events. In the same year, 76.1 percent of children receiving trauma-informed services reported positive functioning at six-month follow-up.

## Primary and Behavioral Health Integration

SAMHSA administers the Primary and Behavioral Health Care Integration (PBHCI) program. The purpose of the program is to improve the physical health status of adults with serious mental illness by supporting communities to coordinate and integrate primary care services into publicly funded community mental health and other community-based behavioral health settings. The program supports community-based behavioral health agencies' efforts to build the partnerships and infrastructure needed to initiate or expand the provision of primary healthcare services for people in treatment for serious mental illness and co-occurring serious mental illness and substance use disorders.

Since September 2009, the program has awarded 94 grants, and 55 percent of awardees are partnering with at least one Federally Qualified Health Center (FQHC). The Health Resources and Services Administration (HRSA) and SAMHSA collaborate to fund a national technical assistance center to help these grantees and FQHCs integrate primary and behavioral health care in both types of settings. This integration of care and agency efforts has resulted in significant physical and behavioral health gains as well as reduced health care expenditures. Some results that are based on grantee-reported outcome measures from February 2010 through January 7, 2013, include:

- Health: The percentage of consumers who rated their overall health as positive increased by 20 percent from baseline to most recent reassessment (N=3737).
- Tobacco Use: The percentage of consumers who reported they were not using tobacco during the past 30 days increased by 6 percent from baseline to most recent reassessment (N=3787).
- Illegal Substance Use: The percentage of consumers who reported that they were not using an illegal substance during the past 30 days increased by 12 percent from baseline to most recent reassessment (N=3568).

## Projects for Assistance in Transition from Homelessness

The Projects for Assistance in Transition from Homelessness (PATH) is a unique program that is specifically authorized to address the needs of individuals with serious mental illness and/or serious mental illness with a co-occurring substance use disorder who are experiencing homelessness or are at risk of homelessness. PATH funds community-based outreach, mental health, substance abuse, case management and other support services, as well as a limited set of housing services to connect homeless individuals to housing services and support them in community housing settings. In the past 5 years, the PATH program has reached approximately 170,000 individuals each year, with an average of about 68,000 of those individuals becoming enrolled in the PATH program each year.

## Youth Violence Prevention

The Safe Schools/Healthy Students program is a unique Federal grant program designed to prevent violence and substance abuse among our nation's youth in schools and communities. Since 1999, this program has been jointly administered and supported by SAMHSA and the Departments of Education and Justice. The Safe Schools/Healthy Students initiative implements an enhanced, coordinated, and comprehensive plan of activities, programs, and services that promote healthy childhood development, prevent violence, and prevent alcohol and drug abuse. A key element of Safe Schools/Healthy Students activities is the expansion of school-based mental health services, as well as referral to treatment to community health providers. SAMHSA is in the process of completing a national cross-site evaluation of Safe Schools/Healthy Students. Preliminary findings include:

- The program has seen significant increases in the number of students who received school-based mental health services, and community-based services.
- Nearly 90 percent of school staff stated that they were better able to detect mental health problems in their students and more than 80 percent of school staff reported that they observed reductions in alcohol and other drug use among their students.
- Over 90 percent of school staff saw reduced violence on school grounds and nearly 80 percent reported that Safe Schools/Healthy Students had reduced violence in their communities.

## PRESIDENT'S *NOW IS THE TIME* INITIATIVES

In addition to the programs discussed above, I would like to share some of the initiatives related to mental health included in the President's proposed plan, *Now is the Time,* which emphasizes early intervention and treatment for young people struggling with mental health problems.

On January 16, 2013, the President announced his plan to ensure that students and young adults receive treatment for mental health issues. These proposals are included in the President's FY 2014 Budget. Specifically, SAMHSA will take a leadership role in initiatives that would:

1. *Reach 750,000 young people through programs to identify mental illness early and refer them to treatment:* To support training for teachers and other adults who regularly interact with students to recognize young people who need help and ensure they are referred to mental health services, the Administration has proposed a new initiative, Project AWARE (Advancing Wellness and Resilience in Education), to provide this training and set up school-community partnerships to promote mental health, and facilitate referrals when needed. This initiative, which will be coordinated with related proposals at the Departments of Justice and Education, has two parts:
   a) *Provide "Mental Health First Aid" training for teachers:* Project AWARE proposes $15 million for training for teachers and other adults who interact with youth to detect and respond to mental illness, including how to encourage adolescents and families experiencing these problems to seek treatment.
   b) *Ensure students with signs of mental illness get referred to treatment:* Project AWARE also proposes $40 million to help states and school districts work with community leaders, law enforcement, mental health agencies, families and youth, and other local organizations to assure students with mental health issues or other behavioral issues are referred to and receive the services they need. This initiative builds on strategies that, for over a decade, have proven to decrease violence in schools and increase the number of students receiving mental health services.
2. Support individuals ages 16 to 25 at high risk for mental illness: The Administration is proposing $25 million for a new initiative, Healthy Transitions, to support innovative state-based strategies to support young people ages 16 to 25 with mental health or substance abuse issues. Efforts to help youth and young adults cannot end when a student leaves high school. Individuals ages 16 to 25 are at high risk for mental illness, substance abuse, and suicide, but they are among

the least likely to seek help. Even those who received services as a child may fall through the cracks when they leave school or turn 18.
3. Train more than 5,000 additional mental health professionals to serve students and young adults: Experts often cite the shortage of skilled mental health service providers as one reason it can be hard to access treatment. To help fill this gap, the Administration is proposing $50 million to train social workers, counselors, psychologists, behavioral health paraprofessionals, marriage and family therapists, nurses, and other mental health professionals. This would allow SAMHSA and HRSA to provide financial support to train more than 5,000 mental health professionals to serve children, adolescents, young adults (including individuals aged 16-25 years old), and their families, in our schools and communities.

As part of his plan to reduce gun violence, President Obama directed Secretaries Sebelius and Duncan to launch a national conversation to increase understanding and awareness about mental health. As part of that effort, on June 3rd, the President and Vice President will host a National Conference on Mental Health.

The conference will bring together people from across the country, including mental health advocates, educators, health care providers, faith leaders, and individuals who have struggled with mental health problems, to discuss how we can all work together to reduce negative attitudes, and help the millions of Americans struggling with mental health problems recognize the importance of reaching out for assistance.

In addition to these initiatives where SAMHSA is taking a leadership role, other offices in the Department of Health and Human Services have been taking steps – as outlined in the President's *Now Is the Time* plan, to expand coverage of mental health services. Additionally, the Department of Education has proposals to *help 8,000 schools create safer and more nurturing school climates and address pervasive violence.*

# ENSURING EFFICIENCIES AND EFFECTIVENESS

## Evaluation, Outcomes and Quality

SAMHSA has a long history of conducting evaluations designed to ascertain information about programs funded with Federal dollars. More recently, SAMHSA has embarked upon a course to enhance the rigor of its evaluations in order to use data to examine the effectiveness of programs, the quality of program implementation, and to better understand how certain interventions or activities influence behavioral health outcomes in communities across the nation. To this end, SAMHSA evaluations are examined to ensure that the methods are appropriate to the evaluation questions and that the right data is collected to inform our understanding of the results of programs.

Recently SAMHSA completed an inventory of all evaluations currently ongoing in the agency.

These evaluations will be closely monitored by evaluation staff and will be strengthened where indicated and possible. These evaluation experts are collaborating with program staff to develop reporting mechanisms to ensure that the data collected in an evaluation are used to inform policies and practices for the future.

SAMHSA has also undertaken to develop a National Behavioral Health Quality Framework (NBHQF), modeled after the National Quality Strategy, to guide behavioral health services and programs throughout the country and to provide a consistent set of validated measures at the payer, practitioner/ program and population levels. The six goals articulated by the NBHQF are: (1) effective services; (2) person-centered care; (3) effective care coordination; (4) use of best practices; (5) safe care; and (6) accessible and high-value care. The draft NBHQF will soon be in its third round of public input with expected release later this year.

## SAMHSA Stewardship

SAMHSA takes its role as a steward of taxpayer dollars seriously. SAMHSA has closely examined its portfolio to find efficiencies and as a result has reduced redundancy or duplication of programs. For example, in 2012, SAMHSA evaluated its contracting process to achieve purchasing efficiencies and leverage similar contracting vehicles.

As a result, SAMHSA consolidated three state technical assistance contracts into a single contract resulting in both programmatic as well as administrative efficiencies. In 2011, several similar consolidations took place. SAMHSA constantly evaluates its programs via review of grantee performance and data collection. Program adjustments, in scope or focus, are directly affected by that data.

**Technical Assistance**

Technical assistance is a key activity provided by SAMHSA in order to ensure that systems, services, and programs are delivered in the most effective and efficient way possible, and to lead the field toward the use of processes and practices that obtain the best outcomes. SAMHSA provides technical assistance not only to its grantees for the implementation of specific grant programs but also to the field at large for system-wide change and enhancement. SAMHSA's technical assistance is provided through staff subject matter experts as well as through a combination of grants and contracts for technical assistance centers and independent organizations that are managed by SAMHSA staff. The provision of technical assistance encompasses a series of strategies, processes, techniques, and activities (e.g., training, consultation, expert guidance, etc.) designed to maximize overall performance and result in improved outcomes. SAMHSA has developed principles to guide its technical assistance efforts. This approach ensures that SAMHSA's technical assistance activities are delivered in the most effective and efficient way possible, leading the behavioral health field toward the use of processes and practices that obtain the highest level of outcomes.

## CONCLUSION

We have made important strides in the prevention, treatment, and recovery supports for mental and addictive disorders. However, much work remains to be done. The Administration continues to advance our work on this important issue and we look forward to continuing to work with the Congress on these efforts.

**End Notes**

[1] Unmet Need for Mental Health Care Among U.S. Children: Variation by Ethnicity and Insurance Status. Sheryl H. Kataoka, M.D., M.S.H.S.; Lily Zhang, M.S.; Kenneth B. Wells, M.D., M.P.H., Am J Psychiatry 2002;159:1548-1555. 10.1176/appi.ajp.159.9.1548.

[2] Substance Abuse and Mental Health Services Administration, Results from the 2011 National Survey on Drug Use and Health: Mental Health Findings, NSDUH Series H-45, HHS Publication No. (SMA) 12-4725. Rockville, MD: Substance Abuse and Mental Health Services Administration, 2012.

[3] Kessler, R. C., Berglund, P., Demler, O., Jin, R., Merikangas, K. R., & Walters, E. E. (2005). Lifetime prevalence and age-of-onset distributions of DSM-IV disorders in the National Comorbidity Survey Replication. Archives of General Psychiatry, 62(6), 593–602.

[4] Pursuant to Section 1912(c) of the Public Health Service Act, SAMHSA's definition of SMI can be found at: http://www.samhsa.gov/healthreform/healthhomes/Definitions SIM SUD 508.pdf.

[5] Pursuant to Section 1911(c) of the Public Health Service Act, SAMHSA's definition of SED can be found at: http://www.samhsa.gov/healthreform/healthhomes/Definitions SIM SUD 508.pdf.

# INDEX

## A

abuse, 28, 33, 34, 36, 98, 99, 101, 108
access, vii, 1, 3, 4, 11, 14, 15, 16, 17, 19, 33, 34, 36, 46, 57, 58, 59, 64, 71, 78, 79, 80, 82, 83, 84, 86, 87, 89, 90, 92, 93, 94, 95, 96, 109
accountability, 59, 93, 94
accounting, 40
accreditation, 23, 101
acupuncture, 79
adaptations, 51
ADHD, 50
administrative support, 89, 92
administrators, 63
adolescents, 28, 35, 36, 59, 99, 105, 108, 109
adulthood, 57, 59
adults, 28, 29, 35, 36, 40, 43, 51, 56, 58, 72, 73, 97, 99, 100, 102, 103, 104, 106, 108, 109
advancements, 31
Afghanistan, 77, 91
age, 14, 28, 29, 35, 37, 53, 57, 59, 64, 74, 99, 112
agencies, viii, 2, 16, 22, 24, 30, 32, 36, 48, 50, 52, 53, 56, 59, 75, 85, 98, 101, 104, 105, 106, 108
aggression, 58
Alaska, 93
alcoholism, 62
alternative medicine, 80
American Psychiatric Association, 12, 21, 74
American Psychological Association, 12, 21, 25
American Samoa, 86
antipsychotic, 60, 95
antisocial behavior, 58
anxiety, 56, 58, 74
anxiety disorder, 74
APA, 21
appointments, 81, 83, 93, 94, 95
arrests, 105
assessment, 46, 83, 95
asylum, 51
audits, 60, 95
authority(s), 5, 33, 74, 75, 92, 104
awareness, 69, 88, 98, 100, 109

## B

barriers, 17, 32, 47, 55, 56, 57, 58, 83, 86, 95
behavioral manifestations, 41
beneficiaries, 23, 62
benefits, 31, 34, 35, 46, 47, 52
bipolar disorder, 40, 43, 56, 57, 73, 74
bipolar illness, 68
bleeding, 49

# Index

blood, 62, 71
blood pressure, 62
Boat, 64
body mass index (BMI), 33, 43
brain, 39, 41, 42, 61
brain activity, 41
breakdown, 68
Bureau of Labor Statistics, 9, 11, 13, 14, 15, 24
businesses, 60

## C

Cabinet, 75
CAM, 80
campaigns, 100
cancer, 47, 56
candidates, 92
cardiac risk, 43
cardiovascular disease, 71
caregivers, 3, 58, 86
CDC, 44
certification, 9, 10, 20, 21, 93
challenges, 24, 45, 46, 47, 85, 90, 91, 96
childhood, 49, 64, 69, 107
children, 23, 27, 28, 29, 35, 36, 49, 56, 57, 58, 59, 60, 73, 97, 98, 99, 100, 102, 103, 104, 105, 109
cholesterol, 71
chronic diseases, 49
chronic illness, 47
cities, 57
citizens, 74, 75
classes, 74
clients, 33, 72, 87
clinical depression, 74
clinical psychologists, viii, 1, 2, 4, 11, 14, 16, 17, 19
clinical psychology, 4, 23
clinical trials, 80
clozapine, 62
collaboration, 30, 33, 52, 59, 78, 88, 104
colleges, 92
common sense, 63, 76

community(s), 8, 27, 28, 29, 30, 31, 32, 36, 45, 48, 54, 55, 56, 57, 58, 59, 60, 61, 62, 63, 68, 71, 73, 74, 75, 78, 79, 82, 83, 84, 86, 87, 88, 89, 90, 98, 103, 104, 105, 106, 107, 108, 109, 110
community service, 105
community-based services, 31, 73, 103, 107
comorbidity, 64
compassion, 56
compensation, 16, 83
complexity, 52, 91
compliance, 104
complications, 71
conference, 109
confidentiality, 87
congress, vii, 1, 22, 23, 24, 25, 60, 63, 96, 98, 102, 111
consensus, vii, 1, 3, 10, 24, 95
consumers, 30, 31, 32, 45, 52, 104, 106
cooperation, 63
coordination, 33, 50, 59, 63, 64, 84, 90, 110
coronary artery disease, 42
cost, vii, 1, 3, 14, 15, 16, 43, 50, 60, 61, 62, 98
cost saving, 61
Council for Community Behavioral Healthcare, v, ix, 67
counseling, 4, 10, 12, 20, 49, 52, 78, 79, 82, 83, 86, 87
cracks, 36, 51, 109
crisis management, 85
cure, 50, 56
curricula, 92

## D

data collection, 81, 100, 110
deaths, 42, 52, 70
decision makers, 3, 99
deinstitutionalization, 46, 49, 54
delusions, 41
Department of Defense, 10, 16, 53, 78
Department of Education, 57, 78, 109
Department of Health and Human Services, viii, 1, 4, 9, 22, 23, 39, 78, 101, 109

Department of Justice, 16, 70
Department of Labor, 24, 52
Department of Veterans Affairs, vi, ix, 16, 22, 25, 77, 80
deployments, 77, 83
depression, 34, 37, 47, 49, 50, 56, 57, 58, 82, 84
despair, 68
detection, 40, 74, 75
diabetes, 37, 47, 62, 71
disability, 31, 40, 46, 50, 51, 52, 70, 83, 100
disaster, 105
discrimination, 28, 33, 67, 68, 69
diseases, 42, 71
disorder, 28, 33, 34, 58, 62, 73, 106
distress, 74, 75, 105
distribution, 14, 43, 101
District of Columbia, 11, 33, 86
DOC, 75
draft, 110
drug abuse, 107
drug interaction, 59
drugs, 50

## E

early warning, 70
education, 5, 10, 15, 20, 32, 52, 69, 81, 88, 90, 92, 100, 105
educational institutions, 23
educational programs, 21
educators, 109
e-mail, 81
emergency, 61, 62, 80
emotional health, 36, 98
emotional problems, 57
employees, 33, 60
employers, 9, 10, 33
employment, 9, 30, 31, 32, 51, 52, 68, 104
employment status, 104
empowerment, 70
encouragement, 96
enhanced service, 89, 92
environment, 58, 86
erosion, 48

evidence, 3, 31, 57, 59, 61, 62, 69, 70, 74, 78, 79, 85, 90, 93, 94, 98, 99
evidence-based practices, 99
Executive Order, 78, 81, 89, 93
exercise, 62
expenditures, 37, 106
expertise, 62, 78, 81, 98
exposure, 105

## F

Facebook, 87
faith, 109
families, 7, 8, 29, 30, 36, 45, 50, 51, 56, 57, 74, 77, 80, 81, 82, 83, 85, 86, 87, 89, 98, 99, 100, 104, 108, 109
family members, 30, 31, 60, 69, 86, 87, 88, 92, 100, 104
family physician, 46
family therapists, viii, 2, 4, 11, 13, 14, 17, 20, 24, 109
family therapy, 4, 8, 20
fear, 85, 100
federal government, vii, viii, 2, 3, 16
federal workforce, 23
financial, 40, 60, 68, 109
financial support, 109
first aid, 61, 74, 75
flexibility, 84, 104
focus groups, 83
food, 62
force, 75
formula, 18
funding, 2, 22, 29, 30, 48, 57, 58, 63, 70, 74, 100, 101, 102, 103, 104
funds, 30, 48, 61, 62, 63, 70, 103, 104, 106

## G

GAO, 24, 94
genes, 42
genomics, 42
Georgia, 68, 70
GI Bill, 92

governments, 5
graduate education, 5
graduate program, 5
grant programs, 103, 111
grants, 16, 32, 53, 71, 100, 106, 111
Great Britain, 51
growth, 16, 24, 29, 31
growth rate, 24
guidance, 6, 63, 80, 91, 100, 101, 111
guidelines, 19, 59, 63, 69, 78
gun control, 54

## H

hallucinations, 41
health care, vii, 1, 2, 3, 4, 14, 15, 22, 24, 31, 33, 34, 37, 40, 45, 46, 47, 48, 49, 50, 53, 56, 58, 60, 62, 63, 64, 74, 75, 77, 78, 79, 82, 83, 84, 85, 89, 91, 92, 93, 95, 96, 98, 101, 106, 109
health care costs, 31, 47, 62, 63
health care professionals, 91
health care system, 53, 58, 77, 95, 98
health condition, 29, 31, 69, 71, 78, 99
health information, 60
health insurance, 33, 34
health practitioners, 24
health problems, 28, 46, 47, 48, 49, 79, 99, 108, 109
health promotion, 34
health services, 16, 24, 29, 30, 33, 34, 45, 47, 78, 81, 84, 89, 92, 95, 98, 104, 108, 110
health status, 32, 106
heart attack, 42
heart disease, 42, 56, 62
hemoglobin, 62
HHS, viii, 1, 4, 14, 16, 23, 24, 36, 37, 43, 71, 78, 89, 111
high blood pressure, 33, 47
high school, 36, 49, 57, 108
higher education, 75
highways, 19
hiring, 78, 81, 89, 91, 92, 93
history, 45, 109

holistic care, 49
homelessness, 51, 106
homes, 55, 85
homicide, 37, 40
hopelessness, 68
hospitalization, 42, 50, 61, 68
host, 109
House, 22, 25, 69, 97
housing, 30, 31, 32, 46, 48, 104, 107
human, 8
hypertension, 47

## I

ideal, 94
identification, 74
illicit substances, 41
improvements, 46, 49, 89, 91
incarceration, 51
income, 43, 58
individuals, vii, 6, 7, 8, 14, 16, 29, 31, 32, 33, 36, 37, 40, 42, 43, 48, 56, 61, 69, 75, 87, 98, 100, 106, 108, 109
industry, 91, 95
infants, 57
infrastructure, 32, 103, 104, 106
injury(s), 40, 83
inmates, 18, 19
institutions, 18, 19, 31, 75, 92
integration, 32, 63, 86, 106
integrity, 95, 104
interface, 59
internship, 6, 8, 93
interpersonal relations, 8
interpersonal relationships, 8
intervention, 40, 42, 57, 74, 81, 82, 87, 105, 108
intervention strategies, 82
investment(s), 4, 31, 51, 52
Iraq, 77
isolation, 64, 68
issues, 29, 34, 35, 36, 53, 58, 61, 75, 83, 85, 93, 108

## J

juvenile justice, 31, 59, 74, 105

## L

labor force, 16
law enforcement, 36, 61, 105, 108
layering, 50
lead, 11, 39, 46, 49, 71, 111
leadership, 35, 48, 59, 89, 92, 108, 109
learning, 50, 90, 100
legislation, vii, 1, 3, 46, 57
level of education, 5
life expectancy, 70
lifestyle changes, 71
lifetime, 29, 40, 99
lithium, 62
living conditions, 105
local government, 29, 101
logistics, 85
longevity, 68
Louisiana, 10

## M

magnitude, 52
major depression, 40
majority, 40, 51, 80
maltreatment, 64
man, 63
management, 6, 9, 30, 49, 56, 64, 68, 69, 70, 72, 73, 83, 85, 94, 104, 106
manic, 68
manic episode, 68
mantle, 48
marketing, 91, 92
marriage, viii, 2, 4, 8, 11, 13, 17, 20, 24, 109
mass, 43
materials, 100
matter, 80, 111
measurement(s), 78, 93, 94, 95
media, 88, 99, 100
median, 14
Medicaid, 29, 31, 34, 35, 48, 51, 52, 53, 58, 59, 60, 61, 62, 63, 64, 69, 70, 71, 72, 73, 101, 103
medical, 9, 20, 34, 35, 40, 42, 46, 47, 48, 51, 70, 79, 80, 81, 82, 83, 84, 94
medical care, 46
Medicare, 4, 16, 22, 23, 29, 35, 47, 53, 62, 63, 69, 71, 101
medication, viii, 2, 4, 6, 7, 8, 15, 49, 62, 69, 95
medicine, 7, 20, 80
membership, 12, 21, 30, 104
mental disorder, 7, 8, 28, 37, 39, 40, 41, 43, 58, 62, 74, 75
mental health professionals, viii, 1, 3, 4, 5, 9, 16, 17, 18, 19, 24, 36, 79, 84, 89, 91, 92, 109
mental health provider, viii, 2, 11, 12, 14, 15, 16, 17, 21, 23, 74, 88
mental illness, 6, 9, 16, 28, 29, 31, 32, 33, 34, 35, 36, 37, 39, 43, 46, 47, 48, 49, 51, 52, 56, 57, 58, 59, 62, 67, 68, 69, 70, 71, 72, 73, 74, 75, 97, 98, 99, 100, 102, 103, 104, 106, 108
metabolic syndrome, 40, 43
methodology, 14, 18
metropolitan areas, 19
Mexico, 10
military, 52, 78, 79, 83, 86, 87
mind-body, 68, 69, 70, 80
minors, 101
misconceptions, 28
mission(s), 23, 27, 28, 39, 86, 91, 97, 98
misunderstanding, 100
misuse, 34
models, 59, 63, 99, 100
mortality, 40, 42, 43, 62, 95
MSW, 7, 23

## N

National Academy of Sciences, 24, 78
National Child Traumatic Stress Network, 105

National Defense Authorization Act, 78
National Institute of Mental Health, v, viii, 39, 68
National Institutes of Health, 39
National Research Council, 37, 64
National Strategy, 53
National Survey, 28, 37, 43, 71, 99, 111
NCS, 64
negative attitudes, 36, 109
neglect, 76
neuroimaging, 42
New York State Office of Mental Health, v, viii, 45, 52
next generation, 46
NHANES, 43
North America, 42
nurses, viii, 2, 3, 4, 6, 9, 10, 11, 13, 14, 62, 64, 71, 109
nursing, 4, 5, 8, 10, 20

## O

Obama, 78
obesity, 43
obstacles, 48
officials, 48
openness, 63
Operation Enduring Freedom, 79
Operation Iraqi Freedom, 79
operations, 91
opportunities, 28, 33, 46, 48, 49, 53, 55, 84, 93, 100
osteopathy, 20
outpatient, 18, 61, 70, 79, 82, 84, 94, 95
outreach, 78, 82, 83, 86, 88, 91, 92, 106
oversight, vii, 1, 3, 94, 95
overweight, 33, 43

## P

pain, 56, 82
paranoia, 41
parenting, 58, 85
parents, 36, 49, 58

parity, 34, 35, 48
parole, 75
participants, 80
patient care, 19, 20
peer support, 3, 67, 68, 69, 70, 72, 82, 93
performance measurement, 93
permit, 74
personal computers, 85
physical health, 31, 32, 61, 62, 70, 74, 75, 106
physicians, 3, 6, 10, 24, 101
pipeline, 91, 92, 93
policy, vii, viii, 1, 2, 3, 15, 16, 24, 33, 45, 46, 75, 84, 100
policy initiative, viii, 2, 15
policy issues, 15
policy makers, viii, 2, 15, 16
population, 16, 17, 18, 19, 23, 24, 28, 37, 40, 41, 56, 62, 81, 87, 91, 95, 110
population group, 16, 17, 18
population size, 16
portfolio, 103, 110
post-traumatic stress disorder, 78
poverty, 51, 52
preschool, 56
prescription drugs, 29
president, 27, 29, 30, 31, 35, 45, 50, 56, 61, 64, 75, 76, 78, 81, 92, 107, 108, 109
President Obama, 92, 109
prevention, 29, 30, 31, 34, 40, 52, 53, 56, 75, 78, 80, 81, 88, 90, 100, 101, 102, 111
principles, 86, 111
private practice, 14
private sector, 51
problem drinking, 84
problem-solving, 85
prodrome, 41
professionals, viii, 2, 4, 16, 17, 19, 36, 61, 71, 85, 92, 100, 109
profit, 18, 60, 85
prognosis, 53, 68
program staff, 110
programming, 52
project, 41, 53
protective factors, 57

# Index

prototype, 91
provider types, vii, viii, 1, 2, 3, 4, 5, 6, 9, 11, 13, 15, 16
psychiatric illness, 62
psychiatrist(s), viii, 1, 2, 4, 6, 9, 11, 12, 17, 18, 19, 20, 47, 58, 64, 69, 91
psychiatry, 4, 7, 9, 10, 20, 92
psychologist(s), viii, 2, 4, 10, 11, 12, 14, 20, 25, 36, 91, 109
psychology, 7, 10, 20, 23, 25, 92
psychosis, 41, 42, 43, 55
psychosocial interventions, viii, 2, 5, 15
psychotherapy, 90
psychotic symptoms, 41
PTSD, 74, 78, 79, 80, 82, 84, 85, 86, 88
public awareness, 69, 87, 88, 100
public education, 67, 69, 100
public health, 4, 24, 34, 39, 52, 70, 74, 75, 89
Public Health Service Act, 112
public officials, 89
Puerto Rico, 86

## Q

qualifications, 5
quality improvement, 60, 78
quality of life, 70, 84, 95

## R

race, 14
reality, 41
recession, 48
recommendations, 47, 80, 90, 91, 94
recovery, 28, 31, 48, 51, 56, 67, 68, 69, 70, 71, 78, 79, 84, 85, 87, 90, 97, 99, 101, 102, 103, 111
recruiting, 25, 80
redundancy, 110
reengineering, 93
reform, 14, 28, 48, 49, 53, 99
Registry, 99
regulations, 60, 101

regulatory framework, 104
rehabilitation, 4, 30, 48, 103
relevance, 23
reliability, 95
replication, 64
requirements, viii, 2, 3, 4, 5, 6, 9, 10, 14, 15, 23, 34, 35
researchers, 12, 42, 64, 99
resilience, 32, 85, 97, 98
resources, 19, 21, 25, 47, 48, 74, 87, 88, 89, 92, 93, 96, 98, 105
response, 61, 82, 83, 89, 90, 94
restrictions, 63
risk(s), 33, 36, 40, 41, 42, 43, 53, 57, 59, 64, 71, 81, 82, 84, 87, 97, 102, 106, 108
risk factors, 40, 43, 57, 71, 81
risk management, 64
rotations, 7
rowing, 68
rural areas, 58, 78, 82, 91
rural schools, 57

## S

safety, 46, 48, 55, 56, 57, 61, 80
SAMHSA, vi, 22, 23, 24, 27, 28, 29, 30, 31, 32, 33, 34, 35, 53, 57, 58, 62, 67, 70, 97, 98, 99, 100, 101, 102, 103, 104, 105, 106, 107, 108, 109, 110, 111, 112
schizophrenia, 40, 41, 42, 43, 44, 50, 57, 62, 73, 95
scholarship, 92
school, 4, 6, 9, 11, 12, 14, 23, 29, 36, 49, 50, 51, 56, 57, 58, 59, 75, 92, 105, 107, 108, 109
school climate, 109
school failure, 49
school psychology, 4
science, 34, 53, 92, 100
scientific understanding, 56
scope, 3, 4, 6, 9, 10, 23, 39, 51, 110
security, 18
SED, 29, 104, 112
self-employed, 11, 12, 13, 14, 15
self-image, 68

Senate, 22, 27, 39, 45, 55, 67, 69, 73, 76, 77
senses, 70
sensitivity, 83, 84
September 11, 77
service organizations, 73
service provider, 36, 109
sex, 14, 43
shortage, 16, 18, 23, 36, 58, 109
showing, 49
side effects, 50, 71
signs, 36, 68, 69, 70, 74, 88, 100, 108
sleep disorders, 82
smoking, 62, 71, 85
smoking cessation, 85
social network, 68
social security, 31, 35, 51, 52
Social Security Administration, 51
social support, 70
social support network, 70
social workers, viii, 2, 4, 11, 13, 14, 16, 17, 20, 24, 36, 109
society, 50, 68
socioeconomic status, 28
solution, 46, 50, 62, 64
special education, 74
specialists, 3, 6, 9, 10, 17, 20, 23, 31, 46, 48, 69, 70, 71, 78, 80
specialization, 20
speech, 75
spending, 29, 31, 62, 101
Spring, 93
SSI, 51
stabilization, 30, 104
staff members, 79, 87
staffing, 16, 78, 83, 90, 91, 94, 95
stakeholders, 89, 91, 98, 99
state(s), viii, 2, 3, 5, 6, 9, 10, 11, 13, 14, 21, 24, 27, 37, 39, 45, 46, 48, 51, 52, 53, 55, 59, 60, 61, 62, 63, 69, 70, 72, 73, 74, 75, 81, 82, 86, 93, 98, 100, 101, 103, 104, 108, 110
state laws, 3, 9
stigma, 47, 67, 68, 69, 84, 85, 87
stress, 68
structural changes, 32
structure, 42
subscribers, 79
substance abuse, 13, 24, 28, 29, 30, 33, 34, 36, 41, 57, 58, 59, 63, 67, 69, 70, 89, 98, 99, 100, 101, 106, 107, 108
Substance Abuse and Mental Health Services Administration (SAMHSA), 4, 11, 22, 23, 24, 27, 53, 68, 71, 97
substance use, 28, 29, 31, 32, 33, 34, 35, 58, 62, 68, 73, 79, 82, 95, 97, 98, 99, 100, 106
substance use disorders, 28, 29, 31, 34, 82, 99, 100
SUD, 80, 112
suicide, 36, 37, 40, 49, 52, 53, 56, 68, 78, 80, 81, 82, 87, 88, 95, 105, 108
suicide attempts, 105
suicide rate, 81
supervision, 19, 60
support services, 48, 101, 102, 103, 106
support staff, 91
surveillance, 98, 99, 100
sustainability, 58, 63
Switzerland, 43
symptoms, 28, 41, 42, 50, 68, 69, 70, 74, 79, 82, 85, 99, 100

# T

talk therapy, viii, 2, 5
target, 4, 82, 88, 98
Task Force, 75, 82
teachers, 35, 36, 63, 108
teams, 31, 51, 78, 81, 93
technical assistance, 2, 22, 53, 100, 103, 106, 110, 111
techniques, 74, 111
technology(s), 83, 84, 95
teleconferencing, 85
telephone, 61
testing, 42, 80, 101
testing program, 101
therapist, 20
therapy, 49, 95
thoughts, 105

# Index

threats, 48
tobacco, 32, 101, 106
toddlers, 57
total costs, 47
toxicity, 59
tracks, 23
trainees, 91, 92
training, viii, 2, 3, 4, 7, 8, 9, 10, 15, 16, 35, 49, 61, 62, 70, 74, 75, 79, 81, 91, 92, 93, 100, 103, 105, 108, 111
training programs, viii, 2, 16, 91, 92
trajectory, 41
transformation, 99
transparency, 95
transportation, 19
trauma, 50, 56, 69, 78, 79, 86, 87, 105
traumatic brain injury, 85
traumatic events, 105
traumatic experiences, 57
treatment methods, 80
trial, 43
tuition, 36

## U

U.S. Department of Labor, 9, 11, 15
uniform, 24
uninsured, 58
united, 7, 11, 12, 14, 23, 24, 39, 40, 41, 44, 62, 100
United States, 7, 11, 12, 14, 23, 24, 39, 40, 41, 44, 62, 100
universities, 92
updating, 29, 94

## V

vacancies, 91, 92
variables, 28
variations, 42
vehicles, 110
Vice President, 75, 76, 109
victimization, 43
victims, 28, 41, 105
videos, 87
Vietnam, 88
violence, 28, 37, 41, 107, 108, 109
vision, 64

## W

wages, vii, viii, 1, 2, 3, 14, 16
war, 87
Washington, 12, 13, 23, 24, 37, 64
weight gain, 68, 71
welfare, 105
well-being, 8, 46, 95
wellness, 70, 88
witnesses, 74
workers, 2, 4, 11, 14, 15, 20
workforce, vii, viii, 1, 2, 3, 4, 11, 14, 15, 16, 24, 34, 52, 69, 92, 93
workload, 18
workplace, 101
World Health Organization (WHO), 40, 43

## Y

young adults, 34, 35, 36, 52, 108, 109
young people, 35, 36, 49, 50, 108